your pregnancy™
Quick Guide

Twins, Triplets and More

your
pregnancy™
Quick Guide

Twins, Triplets and More

*The book you need to have when
you're having more than one*

Glade B. Curtis, M.D., M.P.H., OB/GYN

Judith Schuler, M.S.

Da Capo
LIFE
LONG

A Member of the Perseus Books Group

Copyright © 2005 by Glade B. Curtis and Judith Schuler

Your Pregnancy is a trademark of Da Capo Press.

Designed by Brent Wilcox
Set in 11.5-point Minion by the Perseus Books Group

Library of Congress Cataloging-in-Publication Data
Curtis, Glade B.
   Your pregnancy quick guide : twins, triplets and more the book you need to have when you're having more than one / Glade B. Curtis, Judith Schuler.
     p.   cm.
   Includes index.
   ISBN 0-7382-1008-0 (pbk. : alk. paper)
   1. Multiple birth—Popular works.   2. Multiple pregnancy—Popular works.
3. Prenatal diagnosis.   I. Schuler, Judith.   II. Title.
   RG696.C87   2005
   618.2'5—dc22

2005006540

ISBN-13 978-0-7382-1008-7

First printing, 2005

Published by Da Capo Press
A Member of the Perseus Books Group
http://www.dacapopress.com

Da Capo Press books are available at special discounts for bulk purchases in the U.S. by corporations, institutions, and other organizations. For more information, please contact the Special Markets Department at the Perseus Books Group, 11 Cambridge Center, Cambridge, MA 02142, or call (800) 255-1514 or (617) 252-5298, or email special.markets@perseusbooks.com.

1 2 3 4 5 6 7 8 9—09 08 07 06 05

This book on multiple pregnancies is not intended to cover every aspect of pregnancy with two or more babies or to cover any one subject in great depth. Many books have been written on the subject of pregnancy with multiples.

Our intent with this book is to give you an overview of how a multiple pregnancy is different from a pregnancy with one baby. We hope that with this information at hand, you will be able to discuss and to plan for your particular situation with your physician and other healthcare workers involved in your pregnancy. We believe that, armed with knowledge and understanding, you will be able to proceed with your pregnancy, to the birth of your babies, better prepared for the incredible journey you are undertaking.

Find It Fast!

Giving Birth to More than One Baby

A multiple pregnancy nearly always surprises expectant parents. However, because of today's advanced testing techniques, especially ultrasound, most couples know they're going to have more than one baby early enough to prepare for their arrivals.

Having more than one baby seems more common today. You may have read about multiple births in the newspapers and magazines, and you hear about it on TV and the radio. You may have friends and family members who have given birth to multiples.

The rate of multiple births has increased greatly in the last 25 years. Recent statistics show that in 1 year in the United States, 132,535 births were multiple births. Of that number, 125,134 were births of twins, 6898 were triplets, 434 were quadruplets and 69 were quintuplets or more.

Between 1980 and 1997, the number of twins born increased by nearly 75%. Births involving three or more babies increased five times! Today, over 3% of all births are multiple births—95% of those are twin births. For every 1000 births, 33 are births of multiples (including twins and more). If you are expecting more than one baby, you're not alone!

When talking about pregnancies of more than one baby, in most cases we refer to twins. The chance of a twin pregnancy is more likely than pregnancy with triplets, quadruplets or quintuplets (or even more!). However, some women are giving birth to more babies than we could have imagined not long ago. Today, we are also experiencing more triplet and higher-order births. A triplet birth is not very common; it happens about once in every 7000 deliveries. (Dr. Curtis has been fortunate to deliver two sets of triplets in his medical career.) Quadruplets are born once in every 725,000 births; quintuplets once in every 47 million births!

No matter how it occurs, being pregnant with two or more babies can affect you in many ways. In this book, we discuss how your pregnancy will be different and the types of adjustments you may be required to make. These changes and adjustments may be necessary for your health and the health of your babies. If you are expecting two or more babies, you will visit your doctor more often. Work closely with your doctor and other health-care professionals to help ensure your pregnancy is healthy and safe.

You and your partner may be in shock when you learn you have more than one baby on the way. It's a normal reaction. Eventually the joy of expecting your babies may help offset the apprehension and responsibility you may feel.

You will also need to plan carefully for delivery and care of the babies after you go home. Read the following pages for information on the many different issues surrounding pregnancy with multiples.

Frequency of Multiple Births

The frequency of multiple births is increasing and has been since 1980. Today, it's not uncommon for a friend or sister to tell you she's expecting more than one baby. If you're reading this book, you're probably expecting multiples, too! Besides luck, there are various factors that affect whether you will be one of the fortunate ones who gives birth to more than one baby.

- The frequency of twins depends on the type of twins. *Identical twins* occur about once in every 250 births around the world. This type of twin formation appears not to be influenced by age, race, heredity, number of pregnancies or medications taken for infertility (fertility drugs).
- The incidence of *fraternal twins,* however, *is* influenced by race, heredity, maternal age, the number of

previous pregnancies, and the use of fertility drugs and assisted-reproductive techniques.

- The frequency of multiple fetuses varies among different races. Twins occur in 1 out of every 100 pregnancies in white women compared to 1 out of every 79 pregnancies in black women. Certain areas of Africa have an incredibly high frequency of twins. In some places, twins occur once in every 20 births. Hispanic women also have a slightly higher number of twin births than white women. The occurrence of twins among Asians is less common—about 1 in every 150 births.

- The occurrence of twins in Japan is only 6 per 1000 births, while in Nigeria that rate is over 7 times as great—in Nigeria, fraternal twins are born at a rate of 45 per 1000 babies.

- Heredity plays a part in the occurrence of twins. In one study of fraternal twins, the chance of a female twin giving birth to a set of twins herself was about 1 in 58 births.

- The incidence of twin births can run in families, on the *mother's* side. One study showed that if a woman is the daughter of a twin, she also has a higher chance of having twins. Another study reported that 1 out of 24 (4%) women who had given birth to twins was also a twin, but only 1 out of 60 (1.7%;

about the national average) of the men who had fathered a set of twins was a twin.

- In addition, if you have already given birth to a set of fraternal twins, your chance of having another set of twins quadruples!
- Other reasons for multiple fetuses include:
  - ~ the use of fertility drugs
  - ~ the use of in-vitro fertilization
  - ~ women having babies later in life
  - ~ having more children
  - ~ being very tall or obese
  - ~ you recently discontinued oral contraception
  - ~ taking more folic acid
- Studies have shown that the twin birth rate for women who took folic acid can be as high as double the rate of women who did not take folic acid. It will be interesting in the future to see if the birth rate of twins increases in the United States now that folic acid is added to so many foods on the market.
- Assisted-reproductive technologies (ART) account for nearly 65% of all multiple births. These technologies include ovarian hyperstimulation with insemination, superovulation and in-vitro fertilization. Over 55% of births resulting from assisted-reproductive techniques were multiples.

- We have known for a long time that fertility drugs increase the chance of multiple pregnancies. Several different medications are used to treat infertility. Each one affects a woman's chances of conceiving more than one fetus to a different degree.

- One of the more common medications used to treat infertility is clomiphene (Clomid). It increases the chances of twin fetuses somewhat less than other fertility medications, but an increased chance still exists.

- Twins are also more common in pregnancies that result from implantation of more than one embryo with in-vitro fertilization. This results when several fertilized eggs are placed in a woman's uterus in the hope that at least one will implant. Because in-vitro fertilization procedures are becoming more successful, some medical professionals are calling for implantation of fewer embryos.

- Today, some medical experts support the use of procedures that improve the chance of a woman having a successful pregnancy and a healthy baby. Two procedures that are used for this purpose are *multifetal pregnancy reduction* and *selective termination*. Their use is controversial.

- Multifetal pregnancy reduction is used to improve the chances of survival in pregnancies with three or

The Good, the Bad and the Snuggly

"I was very nervous during my pregnancy with my twins. Everyone kept telling me that twins are born early, and they have a lot of problems because they're premature. I watched my weight while I was pregnant and gained about 42 pounds altogether. I rested a lot, and I ate a healthy diet and took all the vitamins and supplements my doctor told me to. The result? I carried my two little boys until 38 weeks of pregnancy—they were born healthy, with no problems. They were fairly good sized—6 pounds, 2 ounces, and 6 pounds, 7 ounces! I was able to take them home in a few days, once they were stable." —*Margie*

more fetuses that result from ART. It is usually performed in the first trimester, between 10 and 13 weeks of pregnancy.

- Using ultrasound guidance, chemicals are injected into the fetuses selected for reduction. In most cases, the pregnancy is reduced to two babies (twins) to increase the chance of the babies' survival.
- Selective termination refers to termination of one or more fetuses with abnormalities, with the continuation of pregnancy for the other fetus or fetuses.
- Abnormal fetuses are identified by ultrasound or amniocentesis. This procedure is performed the same way as a multifetal pregnancy reduction, described above.

- Because abnormalities may not be identified until later in pregnancy, this procedure may not be performed until the second trimester.
- Women having babies later in life is another reason for multiple fetuses. We know that being an older mother accounts for nearly 35% of all multiple births.
- Age 30 seems to be the magic age beyond which the number of multiple births increases. Over 70% of all multiple births are to women over age 30.
- In the United States, the highest number of multiple births occurs in women over 40; the next highest group is women between the ages of 30 and 39.
- The increase in multiple births among older women has been attributed to higher levels of gonadotropins, the hormones that stimulate the maturation and release of eggs.
- As a woman ages, the level of gonadotropin increases, and she is more likely to produce two or more eggs during one menstrual cycle. Most twin births in older women are fraternal twins (babies born from two different eggs).
- Having more children (or pregnancies) can also result in more than one baby. This is true in all populations and may be related to the mother's age and female hormone changes.

- Some families are more blessed than others. In one case we know of personally, a woman had three single births. Her fourth pregnancy was twins, and her fifth pregnancy was triplets! She and her husband decided on another pregnancy—they were surprised (and probably relieved) when the sixth pregnancy resulted in only one baby.

Identical Twins and Fraternal Twins

Twin fetuses usually result (over 65% of the time) from the fertilization of two separate eggs; each baby has his or her own placenta and amniotic sac. These are called *dizygotic* (two zygotes) *twins* or *fraternal twins.* With fraternal twins, you can have a boy and a girl. About 33% of the time, twins come from a single egg that divides into two similar structures. Each has the potential of developing into a separate individual. These are known as *monozygotic* (one zygote) *twins* or *identical twins.* Identical twins are not always identical. It is possible for fraternal twins to appear more alike than identical twins!

- A multiple pregnancy occurs when a single egg divides after fertilization or when more than one egg is fertilized.
- Monozygotic (identical) twins, from one egg, occur about once in every 250 births around the world.

- Dizygotic (fraternal) twins, from two eggs, occur in 1 out of every 100 births. These rates vary for different races and areas of the world.
- Pregnancy with twins as a result of a fertility treatment most often results in fraternal twins.
- In some cases of higher-number fetuses, a pregnancy can result in fraternal *and* identical twins, when more than one egg is fertilized (dizygotic twins) and, in addition, one of the eggs divides (monozygotic twins).
- The percentage of male fetuses decreases slightly as the number of fetuses in the pregnancy increases. In other words, as the number of babies a woman carries increases, her chances of having more girls than boys also increase.
- For singleton pregnancies, the percentage of males born in the United States is 51.6%. For twins, it is 50.9%, for triplets 49.5% and for quadruplets 46.5%.
- Either or both of the fertilization processes may be involved when more than two fetuses are formed. What we mean by that is triplets may result from fertilization of one, two or three eggs, and quadruplets may result from fertilization of one, two, three or four eggs.
- With monozygotic (identical) twins, division of the fertilized egg occurs between the first few days and about day 8.

- If division of the egg occurs after 8 days, the result can be twins that are connected, called *conjoined twins*. (Conjoined twins used to be called *Siamese twins*.) These babies may share important internal organs, such as the heart, lungs or liver. Fortunately this is a rare occurrence.
- Monozygotic twins may face additional risks. There is a 15% chance monozygotic twins will develop a serious problem called *twin-to-twin transfusion syndrome*. With this condition, there is one placenta; however, one baby gets too much blood flow and the other too little. Research is being done about the problem, and strides are being made in prenatal treatment.
- Research has shown that just because there are two placentas, it doesn't mean twins are dizygotic; nearly 35% of all monozygotic twins have two placentas.
- With monozygotic twins, there is a chance that several different types of diseases may occur in both twins during their lifetimes. This is less likely to happen with dizygotic twins.
- It may be important later in life for your multiples to know whether they were monozygotic or dizygotic, due to health concerns. Before delivery, tell your doctor you would like to have the placenta(s) examined (with a pathology exam) so you will know whether

your babies were monozygotic or dizygotic. It may be valuable information in the future.

Discovering You're Carrying More than One Baby

Diagnosis of twins was more difficult before ultrasound was available. See the discussion of *Ultrasound* that begins on page 47. Today, it is uncommon to discover twin pregnancies just by hearing two heartbeats.

- Most multiple fetuses are discovered during pregnancy, not at the time of delivery. Today, it is uncommon for parents to be surprised by the birth of a second baby.
- A doctor usually discovers a woman is carrying more than one baby because of various signs, including a larger-than-expected uterus, more severe nausea and vomiting, and more than one fetal heartbeat.
- Measuring and examining your abdomen during pregnancy is important. Usually a twin pregnancy is found because you are too big and growth seems too fast for a single pregnancy.
- Multiple pregnancy may also be suspected if you have severe morning sickness, which may also last longer than normal.

- Ultrasound examination is the best way to tell if you are carrying more than one baby.
- When a doctor suspects a woman is carrying more than one baby, an ultrasound is usually ordered. An ultrasound exam almost always detects a multiple pregnancy.

When a Multiple Pregnancy Isn't a Multiple Pregnancy

The occurrence of twins is probably more common than we know. Some women are told early in pregnancy they are carrying twins only to discover later they are carrying only one baby. What happened?

- In some cases, an early ultrasound exam reveals two babies, but later ultrasounds of the same woman show one baby has disappeared, but the other baby is OK.
- Sometimes referred to as the *vanishing twin,* researchers believe one of the fetuses dies and is absorbed by the mother's body. It actually occurs in about 20% of all twin pregnancies.
- We are unsure why it occurs, but research indicates it may be because of a small gestational sac or a small fetus.
- Vanishing twin is one reason many doctors prefer not to predict a twin birth before 10 weeks of preg-

The Good, the Bad and the Snuggly

"Everyone told me to try to get my babies on the same schedule for feeding and sleep, so I worked hard to do it. The same sleeping schedule was great—when the girls slept, I could nap or rest, too. But being on the same feeding schedule was the pits sometimes. They'd both wake up about the same time, ravenous and wanting to be fed *now!* It was hard to listen to one scream while I fed the other one. At times, I'd find myself kneeling on the floor, with both babies in their infant seats, trying to hold a bottle for each of them. The really hard part was burping them afterward!" —*Millie*

nancy. Parents who are informed of twins early in pregnancy may be distraught to learn later that one of the babies will not be born.

- Loss of one twin after the first trimester is called *intrauterine fetal demise (IUFD)*.

Increased Risks of Complications Associated with a Multiple Pregnancy

When you are pregnant with more than one baby, your risk of problems and complications increases. These may be minimized and possibly avoided with good prenatal care and careful attention to your health. In this section, we discuss the more common problems women may experience when they are expecting multiples.

- Possible pregnancy problems include:
  - ~ increased miscarriage
  - ~ fetal death
  - ~ fetal malformations
  - ~ low birth weight or fetal growth restriction
  - ~ pre-eclampsia
  - ~ twin-to-twin transfusion syndrome
  - ~ maternal anemia
  - ~ problems with the placenta
  - ~ maternal bleeding or hemorrhage
  - ~ problems with the umbilical cords
  - ~ hydramnios or polyhydramnios
  - ~ labor complicated by breech or transverse presentation
  - ~ premature labor
  - ~ premature delivery
- One way to reduce risks is to take very good care of yourself during pregnancy.
- Pay strict attention to your eating plan; eat wisely and nutritiously for all of you.
- Extra rest is essential. Most women who are expecting multiples need at least 2 hours of rest during each day.

- When you are pregnant with more than one baby, you are monitored more closely during pregnancy. You will probably have more frequent checkups, and more tests may be ordered for you.
- Beginning in your 20th week, you will probably visit your doctor every other week until the 30th week. Then you may be seen once a week until delivery.
- You may have ultrasound more frequently to monitor the babies' growth.
- Your blood pressure is monitored very closely to check for pre-eclampsia, which is twice as common in multiple pregnancies.
- One of the biggest concerns with multiple pregnancies is premature delivery. As the number of fetuses increases, the length of gestation and individual birth weight decreases, although this is not true in every case. See the discussion of *Premature Birth* beginning on page 107.
- One of the main goals in dealing with multiple fetuses is to continue the pregnancy as long as possible to avoid premature delivery.
- This may best be accomplished by bed rest. See the discussion of *Bed Rest* on page 70.
- If you are on bed rest, you may not be able to carry on with your regular activities, such as going to

work. If your doctor recommends bed rest, follow his or her advice.

- Some researchers believe use of a *tocolytic agent* (medication to stop labor), such as ritodrine, is critical in preventing premature delivery. These agents are used to relax the uterus to stop premature labor or to keep you from going into premature labor.
- During your pregnancy, follow your doctor's instructions closely. Every day and every week you're able to keep the babies inside you are days or weeks you won't have to visit them in an intensive-care nursery while they grow, develop and finish maturing.

If You Have Questions

- If you feel uncomfortable or have questions, don't be afraid to ask for help.
- Call your doctor to discuss your concerns.
- Although you may believe it's easier to get advice or information from family members or friends, *don't* rely on them for medical advice.
- Your doctor has probably dealt with similar situations many times. The answers he or she gives you will be right for your particular pregnancy.

Warning Signs

If you experience any of the following signs or symptoms, call your doctor immediately. General warning signs include:

- vaginal bleeding
- severe swelling of the face or fingers
- severe abdominal pain
- loss of fluid from the vagina (usually a gushing of fluid but sometimes a trickle or a continual wetness)
- a big change in the movement of the babies or a lack of fetal movement
- high fever—higher than 101.6F
- chills
- severe vomiting or an inability to keep food or liquids down
- blurred vision
- painful urination
- a headache that won't go away or a severe headache
- an injury or accident that hurts you or gives you concern about the well-being of your pregnancy, such as a fall or an automobile accident

Intrauterine-Growth Restriction (IUGR)

Intrauterine-growth restriction (IUGR) means a fetus is small for its gestational age. By definition, its birth weight is below the 10th percentile (in the lowest 10%) for the baby's gestational age. This means 9 out of 10 babies of normal growth are larger.

- When due dates are correct and the pregnancy is as far along as expected—and fetal weight falls below the 10th percentile—it's a cause for concern.
- Growth-restricted infants have a higher rate of death and injury than infants in the normal-weight range.
- Diagnosing IUGR can be difficult. One reason your doctor measures you at each visit is to see how your uterus and babies are growing.
- When a problem occurs, it may be found by measuring the uterus over a period of time and finding little or no change, especially with a multiple pregnancy.
- Diagnosis of IUGR is one important reason to keep all your prenatal appointments. You may not like being weighed and measured at every appointment, but it helps your doctor see that your pregnancy is growing and your babies are getting bigger.
- Intrauterine-growth restriction can be diagnosed or confirmed by ultrasound. Ultrasound may also be used to assure the babies are healthy and no malformations exist that must be taken care of at birth.
- If IUGR is diagnosed, avoid doing anything that could make it worse. Be sure you gain enough weight. Stop smoking. Studies show that smokers who didn't gain at least ½ pound a week with a multiple

pregnancy had the highest risk of IUGR. Improve your nutrition. Stop using drugs and alcohol.

- Bed rest is another treatment; see the discussion of *Bed Rest* that begins on page 70.
- Resting on your side enables the babies to receive the best blood flow, and better blood flow is the best chance they have to improve growth.
- If maternal disease causes IUGR, treatment involves improving the mother's general health.
- Babies with intrauterine-growth restriction are at greater risk of dying before delivery. Babies may need to be delivered before they are full term.
- Infants with IUGR may not tolerate labor well; a C-section is more likely because of fetal stress. The babies may be safer outside the uterus than inside of it, in some cases.

Causes of IUGR. What causes intrauterine-growth restriction? Below are some conditions that increase the chance of intrauterine-growth restriction or small fetuses.

- First of all, carrying more than one baby may be a cause of IUGR. There is only so much room inside a woman's uterus, and being pregnant with more than one baby restricts the space available for each one. Thus, babies may be growth restricted.

The Good, the Bad and the Snuggly

"I was expecting triplets in December. My sister-in-law was getting married in August, so I went to her bridal shower. I was huge, even though the babies weren't due for 4 more months. Another pregnant lady sat next to me at the shower, and we got to talking. I asked her when her baby was due—she told me in 5 weeks. She was pretty good sized, but I had her beat. When she asked me when my baby was due, I said December. She couldn't believe it. However, when I explained we were expecting 'numbers two, three and four,' she laughed and said she was glad it was me and not her. I was glad, too." —*Vicki*

- Smoking and other tobacco use can inhibit fetal growth. The more cigarettes a woman smokes, the greater the impairment and the smaller the babies.
- Eating a poor diet during your pregnancy can cause problems.
- Restricting normal weight gain (dieting) during pregnancy may be a factor. Research indicates that when calories are restricted, IUGR may result.
- Pre-eclampsia and high blood pressure (hypertension) can have a marked effect on fetal growth.
- Cytomegalovirus, rubella and other infections may also cause restricted fetal growth.
- Maternal anemia may be a cause of intrauterine-growth restriction.

- Women who live at high altitudes are more likely to have babies who weigh less than those born to women who live at lower altitudes.
- Alcoholism and drug use can cause smaller-than-normal babies. Kidney disease may also be a factor.
- A malformed or abnormal fetus may also be smaller, especially when chromosomal abnormalities are present.

Pregnancy-Induced High Blood Pressure (Hypertension; PIH)

Pregnancy-induced hypertension (high blood pressure), also called *PIH*, occurs *only* during pregnancy. About one pregnant woman in 10 experiences the condition. Most who are hypertensive during pregnancy do not have high blood pressure when they are not pregnant.

- With hypertension of pregnancy, the systolic pressure (the first or top number) increases to higher than 140ml of mercury or a rise of 30ml of mercury over your beginning blood pressure.
- A diastolic reading (the second or bottom number) of over 90, or a rise of 15ml of mercury, also indicates a problem.
- An example is a woman whose blood pressure at the beginning of pregnancy is 100/60. Later in preg-

nancy, it is 133/94. This indicates she may be developing PIH.

- Your blood pressure is important during pregnancy because blood vessels in the uterus supply the placenta with nutrients and oxygen for the developing babies.

- High blood pressure constricts uterine blood vessels, which can slow the passage of nutrients and oxygen from the mother to the placenta to the babies, which slows fetal development.

- Hypertension increases the risk of placental abruption (separation of the placenta from the wall of the uterus before delivery). This situation can cause heavy bleeding and shock, which are dangerous conditions for you and your babies. See the discussion of *Placental Abruption* that begins on page 31.

- Hypertension has other effects. About 20% of all women who experience chronic hypertension (high blood pressure before pregnancy) develop pre-eclampsia.

- About 25% of the women who develop PIH also develop pre-eclampsia. (By comparison, 6% of women who do not have hypertension during pregnancy develop pre-eclampsia.) A discussion of *Pre-eclampsia* begins on page 33.

- Your doctor can determine if your blood pressure is rising to a serious level by checking it at every prenatal appointment. That's another reason it is so important to keep all of your prenatal appointments.

Gestational Diabetes

Some women develop diabetes only during pregnancy; this is called *gestational diabetes.* Gestational diabetes affects about 10% of all pregnancies. After pregnancy, nearly all women with gestational diabetes return to normal, and the problem disappears. However, more than half of the women who experience diabetes during pregnancy become diabetic later in life. In addition, a woman who develops gestational diabetes in one pregnancy has a good chance of developing it in a subsequent pregnancy.

- Gestational diabetes is triggered when the usual hormone changes of pregnancy, combined with dietary factors, result in higher blood-sugar levels.
- Children of diabetic women are more likely to develop diabetes themselves. Daughters of women who developed gestational diabetes are likely to become diabetic during their own pregnancies. If your mother had gestational diabetes, be sure to share this information with your physician.

- In addition, your own weight at birth (when you were born) may indicate your chances of developing gestational diabetes. One study showed women who were in the *bottom* 10th percentile of weight when they were born were 3 to 4 times more likely to develop gestational diabetes during pregnancy.

- During pregnancy, diabetes can cause several medical complications, including kidney, eye, blood and vascular problems. Any of these can be serious for you and your babies.

- If left untreated, you and your babies will be exposed to a high concentration of sugar in the blood, a condition called *hyperglycemia*. This is not healthy for the fetuses.

- Gestational diabetes may cause *polyhydramnios* (production of excessive amounts of amniotic fluid), which can develop at any time during pregnancy. The condition may cause premature labor because the uterus becomes overdistended.

- If your blood-sugar level is elevated, you may experience more infections during pregnancy. The most common infections involve the kidneys, the bladder, the cervix and the uterus.

- If an expectant mother's blood-sugar levels are high, a baby's insulin output increases in an attempt to process the excess and to re-establish a balance.

However, the baby's insulin can't cross the placenta, back to the mother, so the effort doesn't help balance their shared chemistry. The extra insulin remains in the amniotic sac, and the baby's growth may be exaggerated because of it. In some cases, a baby grows very large. This situation can occur with one baby or with more than one baby.

- After birth, a baby may have very low blood sugar, called *hypoglycemia*, because the baby's body now controls its own blood sugar. Babies are checked for the condition immediately after delivery. If the blood-sugar level is low, the baby may be given some sugar.

- The baby may be born with hyperbilirubenemia (severe jaundice). Some babies with this problem have weak or high-pitched cries, appear shaky and tire quickly. A baby may be unable to nurse well or for long enough to get adequate nutrition, which can affect its growth.

- The best way to treat diabetes developed during pregnancy is for you to eat properly. You may need to see a dietitian.

- Under a typical plan, you eat many small meals a day of lowfat, sugar-free, high-fiber foods. Eating this way enables your body to keep sugar production at a more-constant level.

- Drinking lots of water every day is also very important in this plan.
- If you have gestational diabetes, your blood-sugar level may be tested at office visits. Your doctor may also want you to test it at home.

Anemia during Pregnancy

Anemia is a common problem during pregnancy. If you suffer from anemia, treatment is important for you and your babies. There is a fine balance in your body between the production of blood cells that carry oxygen to the rest of your body and the destruction of these cells. Anemia is the condition in which the number of red blood cells is low. When you are anemic, you have an inadequate number of red blood cells.

- During pregnancy, the number of red blood cells in your bloodstream increases. The amount of plasma (the liquid part of the blood) also increases but at a higher rate.
- Your doctor keeps track of these changes in your blood with a *hematocrit* reading. Your hematocrit is a measure of the percentage of the blood that is red blood cells.
- Your *hemoglobin* level is also tested. Hemoglobin is the protein component of red blood cells.

The Good, the Bad and the Snuggly

"My babies were born 7 weeks premature. I had to have an emergency C-section because one of them was very sick—we didn't think he'd make it. But he did. The hard part was that the twins were in a hospital 65 miles away—a long, arduous trip through the mountains. I was very torn about wanting to be with them all the time and also taking care of my other two sons, ages 4 and 6. I don't know how I did it for the 7 weeks the babies were in the hospital, but I traveled back and forth several times a week. I knew my little boys needed me, but I also knew my big boys did, too. It was one of the best days of my life when I brought my second twin home and we could finally be a family!" —*Heather*

- If you are anemic, your hematocrit is lower than 37 and your hemoglobin is under 12.
- A hematocrit determination is usually made at the first prenatal visit along with other lab work. It may be repeated once or twice during pregnancy. It may be done more often if you have anemia.
- If you are anemic, you won't feel well during pregnancy; you'll tire easily, and you may experience dizziness.
- There is always some blood loss at delivery. If you're anemic when your babies are born, you are at higher risk of needing a blood transfusion after your babies' birth.

- Follow your doctor's advice about diet and supplementation if you suffer from anemia.

Iron-Deficiency Anemia

- The most common type of anemia seen in pregnancy is *iron-deficiency anemia.*
- You want to avoid iron-deficiency anemia because it can increase your risk of premature delivery. You are already at increased risk for this because you are carrying more than one baby.
- During pregnancy, your babies use some of your iron stores. If you have iron-deficiency anemia, your body doesn't have enough iron left to make red blood cells because the babies have used some of your iron for their own blood cells.
- Iron is the most important supplement to take. It is required in almost all pregnancies.
- Most prenatal vitamins contain iron, but it is also available as a supplement.
- If you are unable to take a prenatal vitamin, you may be given 300 to 350mg of ferrous sulphate or ferrous gluconate 2 or 3 times a day.
- Even with supplemental iron, some women develop iron-deficiency anemia during pregnancy. Several factors, some of which you may experience during a pregnancy with multiples, may make a

woman more likely to have this condition in pregnancy, including:

~ poor dietary habits

~ failure to take iron or failure to take a prenatal vitamin containing iron

~ bleeding during pregnancy

~ previous surgery on the stomach or part of the small bowel (making it difficult to absorb an adequate amount of iron before pregnancy)

~ antacid overuse that causes a decrease in iron absorption

- The goal in treating iron-deficiency anemia is to increase the amount of iron you consume. Iron is poorly absorbed through the gastrointestinal tract and must be taken on a daily basis. It can be given as an injection, but it's painful and may stain the skin.

- Side effects of taking iron supplements include nausea and vomiting, with stomach upset. If this occurs, you may have to take a lower dose.

- Taking iron may also cause constipation.

- If you cannot take an oral iron supplement, an increase in dietary iron from foods, such as liver or spinach, may help prevent anemia.

- Ask your doctor for information on what types of foods you should include in your diet.

Placental Abruption

- Placental abruption is premature separation of the placenta from the uterine wall.
- Normally, the placenta does not separate from the uterus until after a baby is delivered. Separation before delivery can be very serious.
- Placental abruption occurs in about 1 in every 200 deliveries.
- The cause of placental abruption is unknown. Certain conditions may increase the chance of its occurrence, including:
  - ~ multiple fetuses
  - ~ physical injury to the mother, as from a car accident
  - ~ a short umbilical cord
  - ~ sudden change in the size of the uterus (from delivery or rupture of membranes)
  - ~ hypertension
  - ~ dietary deficiency
  - ~ a uterine abnormality, such as a band of tissue in the uterus where the placenta cannot attach properly
  - ~ previous surgery on the uterus (removal of fibroids) or D&C for abortion or miscarriage
  - ~ pre-eclampsia

~ uterine fibroids

~ increased maternal age and a higher number of pregnancies

~ cocaine use

- Folic-acid deficiency may play a role in causing placental abruption.

- Expectant mothers who smoke and drink alcohol during pregnancy may be more likely to have placental abruption.

- A woman who has had placental abruption in the past is at an increased risk of having it recur. The rate of recurrence has been estimated to be as high as 10%.

- Separation of the placenta may involve partial or total separation from the uterine wall.

- The situation is most severe when the placenta separates totally from the uterine wall.

- A baby relies entirely on circulation from the placenta. When it separates, the baby cannot receive blood from the umbilical cord, which is attached to the placenta.

- Symptoms of placental abruption can vary a great deal. There may be heavy bleeding from the vagina, or you may experience no bleeding at all.

- Other symptoms can include lower-back pain, tenderness of the uterus or abdomen, and contractions or tightening of the uterus.

- Ultrasound may be helpful in diagnosing this problem, although it does not always provide an exact diagnosis.
- Serious problems, such as shock because of the rapid loss of large quantities of blood, may occur with premature separation of the placenta.
- Blood clotting can also be a problem.
- Treatment of placental abruption varies.
- With heavy bleeding, delivery of the babies may be necessary.
- When bleeding is not heavy, the problem may be treated with a more conservative approach. This depends on whether either fetus is stressed or appears to be in immediate danger.
- Placental abruption is one of the most serious problems related to the second and third trimesters of pregnancy. If you have any symptoms, call your doctor immediately!
- With multiple fetuses, the uterus can get very large, very quickly, which can increase the risk of placental abruption.

Pre-eclampsia

- *Pre-eclampsia* describes a variety of symptoms that occur only during pregnancy or shortly after delivery.

- Symptoms of pre-eclampsia include swelling (edema), protein in the urine (proteinuria), hypertension (high blood pressure) and a change in reflexes (hyperreflexia).
- Other nonspecific, important symptoms of pre-eclampsia include pain under the ribs on the right side, headache, seeing spots or other changes in vision.
- Most pregnant women have some swelling during pregnancy; swelling in the legs does not necessarily mean you have pre-eclampsia.
- It is also possible to have hypertension during pregnancy without having pre-eclampsia.
- The above signs are all warning signs. Report them to your doctor immediately, particularly if you've had blood-pressure problems during pregnancy!
- Laboratory tests include *h*emolysis, *e*levated *l*iver enzymes and *l*ow *p*latelet counts to diagnose HELLP syndrome.
- HELLP syndrome is severe pre-eclampsia and is associated with increased risks for mother and fetus.
- We are not certain what causes pre-eclampsia, but one study shows that women who developed pre-eclampsia had a specific protein present in the cells of their placenta. This protein binds two growth factors that are needed for healthy fetal development. A

The Good, the Bad and the Snuggly

"My quads were born at 28 weeks—they were so small and help-less. All four were put in the NICU immediately; I know the won-derful care they received there saved their lives. The people in the NICU were fantastic—they helped me learn about each baby and encouraged me and other family members to take care of them. The babies were in the hospital for 11 weeks, but the help I re-ceived from the nurses and doctors made me confident that I could take care of my babies once they were all home." —*Angie*

great deal more research needs to be done, but we may be on the right track to treat this serious preg-nancy problem in the future.

- Pre-eclampsia occurs most often during a woman's first pregnancy. Other risk factors include:
  - ~ carrying more than one baby (multiples)
  - ~ pre-eclampsia in a previous pregnancy
  - ~ chronic high blood pressure
  - ~ diabetes, obesity
  - ~ being older
  - ~ being African-American
- Women over 30 years old who are having their first baby are more likely to develop high blood pressure and pre-eclampsia.
- Studies show that more than 50% of all triplet preg-nancies are complicated by pre-eclampsia.

- Some researchers believe that working women may be more likely to develop pre-eclampsia due to job stress.
- Other researchers believe the tendency to develop the problem is genetically inherited.
- If you are in a stressful job situation, discuss it with your physician.
- The goal in treating pre-eclampsia is to avoid eclampsia (seizures). See the discussion below.
- Rapid weight gain, often due to increased water retention, can be a sign of pre-eclampsia or worsening pre-eclampsia.
- Treatment of pre-eclampsia begins with bed rest at home. You may not be able to work or to spend much time on your feet.
- Bed rest allows for the most efficient functioning of your kidneys and the greatest blood flow to the uterus.
- Lie on your side, not on your back. Drink lots of water. Avoid salt, salty foods and foods that contain sodium, which may cause you to retain fluid.
- If you can't rest at home in bed or if symptoms do not improve, you may be admitted to the hospital or your babies may need to be delivered.
- Babies are delivered to avoid seizures in you and for the babies' well-being.

- During labor, pre-eclampsia may be treated with magnesium sulfate. It is given by I.V. to prevent seizures during and after delivery.
- Pre-eclampsia can progress to eclampsia. *Eclampsia* refers to seizures or convulsions in a woman with pre-eclampsia.
- The seizures with pre-eclampsia are not caused by a previous history of epilepsy or a seizure disorder.
- If you think you've had a seizure, call your doctor immediately!
- Eclampsia is treated with medications similar to those prescribed for seizure disorders.
- Women with multiples are more likely to become pre-eclamptic.

Target Weight Gain with Multiples

Weight gain is important with a multiple pregnancy. The target weight gain for women carrying more than one baby is quite a bit higher than that for women carrying one baby.

- You will need to gain more than a woman who is carrying only one baby. The desirable weight gain for women expecting twins is 35 to 45 pounds. For a woman expecting triplets, that weight gain can be as high as 50 to 60 pounds. If you're carrying triplets or more, your doctor can advise you how much weight you should gain during your pregnancy.

- It's important to gain weight in the first half of pregnancy because multiple pregnancies are often shorter than singleton pregnancies.
- If you gain your weight early, it helps in the development of the placenta(s), which may help in its function of passing nutrients to your babies.
- A good goal to set is to gain 24 pounds by 24 weeks with twins, and 34 pounds by 24 weeks with triplets. With a twin pregnancy, this means a gain of about 1 pound a week. With a triplet pregnancy, it is a gain of nearly 1½ pounds a week.
- Studies show that if a woman gains the targeted amount of weight with a multiple pregnancy, her babies are often healthier.
- Usually women who gain the targeted amount of weight during pregnancy lose it after delivery. You don't have to carry the extra weight forever, so don't worry about it now.
- One study showed that women who gained the suggested amount of weight during a twin pregnancy were close to their prepregnant weight 2 years after delivery.

- When you consider the average size of the babies (about 4 to 6 pounds each) and the weight of the placenta(s) (up to 1½ pounds for each), plus the weight of the additional amniotic fluid, you can see where some of your extra weight comes from.

Are You an Older Mother-to-Be?

As discussed earlier, being older may influence whether you have a multiple pregnancy. More women every year are getting pregnant in their 30s or 40s. If you waited to start a family, you are not alone. In the 1980s, births to women in the 35- to 44-year-old age range nearly doubled. First births to women in their 30s in 1990 accounted for about 25% of all births to women in that age group.

- Every day in the United States, nearly 200 women 35 or older give birth to their first child. Researchers believe that in the 21st century, nearly one in every 10 babies will be born to a mother aged 35 or older.
- Most women who become pregnant in their 30s and 40s are in good health. A woman in good physical condition may go through pregnancy as easily as a woman 15 to 20 years younger. An exception— women in a first pregnancy who are over 40 may

encounter more complications than women the same age who have previously had children.

- If you are older, you and your partner may want to consider genetic counseling.
- Genetic counseling brings together a couple and professionals who are trained to deal with the questions and problems associated with the occurrence, or risk of occurrence, of a genetic problem.
- Information about human genetics is applied to a particular couple's situation. Data is interpreted so the couple can understand it and make informed decisions about childbearing.
- As an older pregnant woman, your doctor may see you more often or you may have more tests performed.
- You may be advised to have amniocentesis or chorionic villus sampling (CVS) to determine whether either of your babies will have Down syndrome. This is advisable, even if you would never terminate your pregnancy. Knowing these facts helps you prepare for the birth of your babies.
- You may be watched more closely during pregnancy for signs and symptoms of gestational diabetes or hypertension. Both can be troublesome during pregnancy, but with good medical care, they usually can be handled fairly well.

- You may gain more weight, see stretch marks where there were none before, notice your breasts sag lower and feel a lack of tone in your muscles. Pregnancy and being older can take their toll.
- Because of demands on your time and energy, fatigue may be one of your greatest problems. It's a pregnant woman's most common complaint.
- Rest is essential to your health and to your babies' health. Seize every opportunity to rest and to nap. Don't take on more tasks or new roles. Don't volunteer for a big project at work or anywhere else. Learn to say, "No." You'll feel better!
- Stress can also be a problem. To alleviate feelings of stress, exercise, eat healthfully and get as much rest as possible. Make time for yourself.
- Some women find a pregnancy support group is an excellent way to deal with difficulties they may experience. Check with your doctor for further information.

Tests for the Woman Expecting More than One Baby

If you are carrying more than one baby, your pregnancy will be different from a pregnancy with only one fetus. Even

The Good, the Bad and the Snuggly

"When my babies were born, they had to stay in the hospital for quite a while. My OB-GYN had talked to me about how important it was to breastfeed my babies, especially if they were premature. I was distressed that I couldn't breastfeed my babies—they had to be hooked up to feeding tubes. The lactation specialist I talked to after they were born encouraged me to pump my breast milk and bring it to the hospital for their feedings. I pumped and stored the extra milk. The babies did very well on the pumped breast milk. When I brought them home, neither of them would breastfeed, so I kept pumping. I divided the milk up between the two of them and supplemented with special preemie formula. I did that until they were 8 months old. I think it gave them a good start in life." —*Alicia*

the number of tests you receive, and when you receive them, may be different. In many cases, a screening test is the first indication a woman is carrying more than one baby.

- Some medical experts recommend that if you are at least 32 years old and your doctor determines you are carrying more than one baby, you should be offered chromosome testing, such as amniocentesis or chorionic villus sampling.
- Research indicates there is a slightly higher chance of abnormalities when a woman is carrying two or more babies.

- An abnormal test result does not necessarily indicate the babies have a problem; it alerts the doctor to perform follow-up tests.
- Often with a multiple pregnancy, blood tests are repeated around week 28 and done to check for gestational diabetes.
- Tests can also reveal if a mother-to-be is anemic, which is more common in women carrying multiples.
- Tests may be performed if other problems develop.
- Amniocentesis may be done to check lung maturity in the babies if there is an indication of preterm labor or pre-eclampsia in the mother. Respiratory distress syndrome is a serious complication for multiples who are delivered too early.

Alpha-fetoprotein Test

- The alpha-fetoprotein (AFP) test is a blood test done on a mother-to-be to help the doctor predict problems in her baby.
- The AFP test can detect neural-tube defects, severe kidney or liver disease, esophageal or intestinal blockage, urinary obstruction, fragility of a baby's bones and Down syndrome.

- Alpha-fetoprotein is produced in a baby's liver, and it passes into the mother-to-be's bloodstream in small quantities, where it can be measured.
- The AFP test is usually performed between 16 and 20 weeks of pregnancy.
- Test results must be correlated with the mother's age and weight, and the gestational age of the fetuses.
- A pregnancy with multiple fetuses will cause an elevation in AFP. Sometimes this test is the first clue that a woman is carrying more than one baby.
- If the AFP test detects a possible problem, more-definitive testing is usually ordered.
- The test detects about 25% of the cases of Down syndrome; if Down syndrome is indicated by the AFP test, additional diagnostic tests are usually ordered.
- At this time, the AFP test is not performed on all pregnant women, but it is required in some states.
- If the test is not offered to you, discuss it with your doctor at one of your first prenatal visits.
- An important use of the test is to help a woman decide whether to have amniocentesis. If an AFP test is abnormal, one of the next tests that may be done is amniocentesis.
- One problem with the AFP test is a very high number of false-positive results. This means the results say there is a problem when there isn't one.

- Currently, if 1000 women take an AFP test, 40 test results may come back "abnormal." Of those 40, only one or two women actually have a problem.
- If you have an AFP and the test result is abnormal, don't panic! You will probably have another AFP test, and an ultrasound may also be performed.
- Results from these additional tests should give a clearer answer.
- Be sure you understand what "false-positive" and "false-negative" test results mean. Ask the doctor to explain what each result can mean to you.

Multiple-Marker Screening Tests

- Tests that go beyond alpha-fetoprotein testing are available now to help a doctor determine if a fetus might have Down syndrome and to rule out other problems in a pregnancy.
- These tests are often called *multiple-marker screening tests* and include the triple-screen test and the quad-screen test (discussed below).

The Triple-Screen Test
- The *triple-screen test* helps identify problems during pregnancy using three blood components—alpha-fetoprotein (AFP), human chorionic gonadotropin

(HCG) and unconjugated estriol, a form of estrogen produced by the placenta.

- Abnormal levels of these three blood chemicals can indicate Down syndrome or neural-tube defects.
- The triple-screen test is considered more accurate than the AFP test alone because there are fewer false-positive results with the triple-screen test.
- Higher levels of HCG in your blood, combined with lower levels of AFP and estriol, may indicate a baby has Down syndrome.
- A false-positive test could result from a wrong due date. If you believe you are 16 weeks pregnant, but are actually 18 weeks pregnant, your hormone levels will be off, which could make the test results incorrect.
- Test results may be false-positive if you are carrying more than one baby.
- An ultrasound done between 18 and 20 weeks of pregnancy can often answer questions when a test result is positive.
- If you have a positive test result, your doctor may suggest further testing.

The Quad-Screen Test
- The *quad-screen test* is like the triple-screen but adds a fourth measurement—the blood level of in-

hibin-A, a chemical produced by the ovaries and placenta.

- This fourth measurement raises the sensitivity of the standard triple-screen test in determining if a fetus has Down syndrome.
- It can also predict neural-tube defects, such as spina bifida.
- Measuring the level of inhibin-A increases the detection rate of Down syndrome and lowers the false-positive rate.
- An ultrasound done between 18 and 20 weeks of pregnancy can often answer questions when a test result is positive.
- If you have a positive test result, your doctor may suggest further testing.

Ultrasound

- An ultrasound exam can be one of the most exciting, fun tests you'll have during pregnancy! The terms *ultrasound, sonogram* and *sonography* refer to the same test.
- Many doctors routinely perform ultrasound exams on their pregnant patients, but not every doctor does them with every patient.

- Ultrasound gives a 2-dimensional picture of a developing baby.
- A device emits sound waves, then picks up echoes of those sound waves as they bounce off the baby. A computer then translates them into a picture. This can be compared to radar used by airplanes or ships to create a picture of the terrain under a night sky or on the ocean floor.
- An ultrasound can be done just about any time during pregnancy.
- The test is usually done at certain times in pregnancy to determine specific information. When you have the test, it may be the point at which you learn you're carrying more than one baby!
- Although you might consider ultrasound an enjoyable way to see your babies grow and to find out what sex they are, the test can be very valuable to your doctor for many reasons.
- Ultrasound helps the doctor check for many details of the babies' growth and development. It has also proved very effective in diagnosing some birth defects.
- The test can help the doctor evaluate your pregnancy in many ways, including:
  - ~ finding out how many fetuses there are
  - ~ determining or confirming a due date

The Good, the Bad and the Snuggly

"I was very uncomfortable during my pregnancy with triplets. There just wasn't enough room for all three of them. While I carried them, sometimes it felt like World War III inside of me; they seemed to be battling for space. Nights were the worst. I couldn't lie down, so I slept in a lounge chair for the last 3½ months. It was a glorious day after they were born, when I could finally sleep on my stomach again!" —*Janie*

~ screening for Down syndrome

~ checking babies' growth

~ checking to see if major physical characteristics of the fetuses are normal

~ looking at a fetus's brain, spine, face, major organs or limbs

~ locating the placenta for use with other tests, such as amniocentesis

~ providing information on the condition of the placenta(s), umbilical cord(s) and the amount of amniotic fluid in the uterus

~ identifying IUGR

~ predicting problems with the placenta, such as placenta previa or placental abruption

~ checking on the babies after a mother-to-be falls or has an accident

~ as part of a biophysical profile

- Ultrasound may be combined with other tests. For example, when it is combined with the triple-screen test, the combination of the two tests can better predict Down syndrome and trisomy 18, also referred to as *Edward's syndrome.*
- When you are carrying multiples, you may receive many ultrasounds during your pregnancy. It's one way for your doctor to check on your babies.
- An ultrasound test may be done at a lab or radiology department. In some cases, a doctor or technician will do the test in the office at a visit, if the office has ultrasound equipment.
- Before the test, you may be asked to drink 32 ounces (1 quart) of water; this amount of water makes it easier to see the uterus.
- You will lie on a table, and the doctor or technician (depending on where the test is done) will apply gel to your abdominal area.
- A device called a *transducer* will be passed back and forth across your tummy.
- A picture will be produced on the screen of the ultrasound machine.
- The picture may not make much sense to you at first. It may be very difficult to see details. Ask the technician to help you.

- You may be able to take a picture of the ultrasound image with you when you leave. Or you may be able to have a videotape made while the test is being done. Ask whether you should bring a new, unused video with you to your ultrasound test.

- This test is one your partner will probably enjoy as much as you will. Tell him about it before you schedule one of your tests so he can check his schedule. Then you can share it together.

- When your test is done after 18 weeks, it *may* be possible to determine the sex of your babies, but don't count on it. It is harder to determine the babies' sexes when there are two or more fetuses in the uterus. It can be difficult to get a clear look because of the babies' positions.

- Even if the technician or your doctor makes a prediction as to the sexes of your babies, keep in mind that a prediction by ultrasound is *not* always right.

Some Special Uses of Ultrasound

- Researchers have developed a method that can be used during a routine ultrasound to help predict a baby's chances of having Down syndrome.

- When combined with blood tests (AFP, triple screen, quad screen), ultrasound has been shown to detect Down syndrome in the fetuses of older women (over 35) with a 97.6% accuracy!

- A lesser-used type of ultrasound is called *vaginal probe ultrasound* or *transvaginal sonography*; it can be very helpful in evaluating problems early in pregnancy, such as a possible miscarriage or ectopic pregnancy.
- This type of ultrasound sometimes gives better information earlier in pregnancy than an abdominal ultrasound does.
- If you have an ultrasound exam in the third trimester, your doctor is looking for particular information. Performed later in pregnancy, this test can help your doctor:
  - ~ monitor the growth of multiples
  - ~ evaluate the babies' size
  - ~ determine the cause of vaginal bleeding
  - ~ check for IUGR
  - ~ determine the cause of vaginal or abdominal pain
  - ~ evaluate the babies after an accident or injury to the mother-to-be
  - ~ detect some fetal malformations
  - ~ monitor a high-risk pregnancy
  - ~ measure the amount of amniotic fluid
  - ~ determine maturity of the placenta(s)
  - ~ with amniocentesis, determine fetal lung maturity

    ~ as part of a biophysical profile, provide reassurance of fetal well-being

- In some areas, 3-dimensional ultrasound is being used; however, it is not available everywhere.

- A 3-dimensional ultrasound provides clear, detailed pictures of the fetuses in the womb.

- These pictures are so clear that the image almost looks like a picture taken by a camera.

- For you, the test is almost the same as a regular ultrasound.

- The difference is that computer software "translates" the picture into a 3-D image.

- A 3-D ultrasound is not necessary in most pregnancies.

- At this time, this advanced ultrasound is used when there is suspicion of abnormalities and the doctor wants to take a closer look.

- Doctors have found many uses for 3-D ultrasound, including:
  - ~ improving the measurement of amniotic-fluid volume
  - ~ showing better pictures of the skull
  - ~ helping to evaluate a baby's spine
  - ~ revealing subtle differences with cleft lip and cleft palate problems involving the face, lips, tooth buds, chin, ears, nose and eyes

~ uncovering defects in the abdominal wall, such as herniated loops of the large and small intestines
~ allowing for better evaluation of the placenta(s), which can be very helpful when you're carrying more than one baby
~ helping the doctor see some abnormalities of the umbilical cord, such as a two-vessel cord
~ helping to rule out other birth defects

Amniocentesis

- Amniocentesis is a test that removes amniotic fluid from the amniotic sac for testing. Fluid can be tested for some genetic defects, infections, meconium and fetal lung maturity.
- The good news about amniocentesis is that over 95% of women who have the test learn their babies do *not* have the disorder the test was done for!
- Amniocentesis can identify about 40 fetal abnormalities (out of 400).
- It is usually performed for prenatal evaluation at around 16 weeks of pregnancy. Some doctors now do the test at around 11 or 12 weeks; however, this early use is controversial.
- The test is often used to screen for chromosomal defects, such as Down syndrome, and some specific gene defects, including cystic fibrosis and sickle-cell disease.

- Amniocentesis may also be done to see if the babies of a sensitized Rh-negative woman are having problems.
- Toward the end of a pregnancy, the test may be done to determine if fetal lungs are mature.
- Amniocentesis can also determine a baby's sex. However, the test is not used for this purpose except in cases in which a baby's sex could predict a problem, such as hemophilia or certain types of muscular dystrophy that occur more often in males.
- In some instances, the test is done to check for infections or for meconium in amniotic fluid.
- The test is usually done in a hospital setting, by a physician skilled in doing the procedure.
- Ultrasound locates a pocket of fluid where the fetuses and placenta(s) are not in the way.
- Skin over the mother's abdomen is cleaned and numbed with a local anesthetic.
- A needle is passed through the abdomen into the uterus, and fluid is withdrawn with a syringe.
- About 1 ounce of amniotic fluid is needed to perform tests; if you are carrying twins, fluid is often taken from each sac.
- Rarely, extracted cells do not grow, so the procedure must be repeated. However, don't panic. This situation does *not* mean a fetus has a problem.

The Good, the Bad and the Snuggly

"During my pregnancy with my twins, I had anemia. I guess I didn't pay enough attention to my diet and didn't eat healthfully. My doctor prescribed iron pills, which helped with the anemia. But then I had trouble with constipation. If I ever get pregnant with multiples again, my nutrition plan will be top on my list of priorities!" —*Lori*

- You will probably want your partner or someone else to accompany you to the test to offer moral support and to drive you home when you are finished.
- Although risks are relatively small, there is some risk associated with the procedure, including trauma to the fetuses, trauma to the placenta(s) or umbilical cord(s), infection, miscarriage or premature labor.
- Fetal loss from complications related to amniocentesis is estimated to be between 0.3 and 3%.
- Discuss risks with the doctor before you decide whether you will have the test.

Fetal Fibronectin (fFN) Test

- Fetal fibronectin (fFN) is a protein found in vaginal secretions up to about 20 weeks of pregnancy.
- If a doctor believes a woman may be going into premature labor, he or she may decide to do the fFN

test to see if there is an increased risk for premature delivery.

- There is a lower risk of preterm birth when the test result for fFN is negative after 22 weeks and before 35 weeks of pregnancy.
- A negative fetal fibronectin test is useful in ruling out impending preterm labor.
- A positive test result is less helpful.
- The test is done the same way as a Pap smear is performed.
- A swab of cervical-vaginal secretions is taken from the top of the vagina, behind the cervix.
- Then it is sent to the lab, where it is tested for fFN.
- Results are available within 24 hours.
- If fFN is present after 22 weeks, it indicates increased risk for preterm delivery.
- If it is absent, the risk is low, and the woman probably won't deliver in the next 2 weeks.

Nonstress Test (NST)

- A nonstress test (NST) is a simple, noninvasive procedure done at 32 weeks of pregnancy or later.
- The test is performed in the doctor's office or in the labor-and-delivery department at the hospital.

- It measures fetal well-being by evaluating the response of the fetal heart to movement of the fetus.
- Doctors use the findings from the NST to help them evaluate how well your babies are tolerating life inside the uterus.
- The nonstress test is commonly used in overdue and high-risk pregnancies. A multiple pregnancy is considered high risk.
- While you are lying down, a technician attaches a fetal monitor (Doppler ultrasound) to your abdomen.
- Every time you feel either of your babies move, you push a button to make a mark on a strip of monitor paper. At the same time, the monitor records the baby's heartbeat.
- When a baby moves, its heart rate usually goes up.
- If the babies don't move or if the heart rate does not react to movement, the test is called *nonreactive*.
- When babies don't move, it doesn't necessarily mean there is a problem—they may be sleeping.
- To help make the babies move, you may be given something to eat or drink.
- If the babies still don't move, a buzzer that creates a sound and vibration to wake up the fetuses may be used. This is called *vibration stimulation*.
- In more than 75% of nonreactive tests, the babies are healthy.

- However, a nonreactive test might be a sign a baby is not receiving enough oxygen or is experiencing some other problem.
- In this case, the test will probably be repeated in 24 hours or additional tests will be ordered, including a contraction-stress test or a biophysical profile. See the discussions that follow.
- This test takes from 10 minutes to 45 minutes to complete.
- Your doctor will decide if further action is necessary.

Contraction-Stress Test (CST)

- If the nonstress test is nonreactive (see the discussion above), a contraction-stress test (CST), also called a *stress test,* may be ordered.
- This test measures the response of the fetal heart to mild uterine contractions that mimic labor and gives an indication of how the babies are doing and how well they might tolerate contractions and labor.
- If you had a problem pregnancy in the past or have experienced medical problems during this pregnancy, your doctor may order this test in the last few weeks of pregnancy.
- If you have diabetes and take insulin, your babies may be at some increased risk of problems. In that

situation, the test may be done every week, beginning around 32 weeks.

- In some cases, the doctor may order the nonstress test alone or order both the nonstress test and the contraction-stress test at the same time. (The contraction-stress test is considered more accurate than the nonstress test.)

- A contraction-stress test is usually done in the hospital because it can take an hour or more and occasionally triggers labor.

- Because a CST involves producing contractions, extra care must be taken so the test doesn't lead to premature labor.

- Three contractions must be recorded in about 10 minutes; each contraction must last about 40 seconds.

- The test can last as long as 2 hours.

- A nurse places a monitor on your abdomen to record the fetal heart rates.

- You are attached to an I.V. that dispenses small amounts of the hormone oxytocin to make your uterus contract.

- Or nipple stimulation may be used to make your uterus contract.

- When the uterus contracts, the blood flow to the placenta decreases.

- If a baby is having trouble or the placenta isn't working well, the contractions can decrease the oxygen supply to that baby. This causes the fetal heart rate to drop.
- The babies' heartbeats are monitored for their responses to the contractions.
- The results of the test can be classified as *negative, positive, unsatisfactory* or *equivocal.*
- A negative test is good.
- A positive test is not good.
- Unsatisfactory or equivocal results mean the test was neither positive nor negative.
- Test results can indicate how well a baby might tolerate contractions and labor.
- If a baby doesn't respond well to contractions, it can be a sign of fetal stress.
- A slowed heart rate after a contraction may be a sign of fetal stress.
- The doctor may recommend delivery of the babies, if the CST is not reassuring.
- In other cases, the test may be repeated the next day, or a biophysical profile may be ordered. (See the discussion beginning on page 62.)
- If the test shows no sign of a slowed fetal heart rate, the test result is reassuring.

- Some believe this test is more accurate than the nonstress test in evaluating a baby's well-being.
- In multiple pregnancies, it can be difficult to perform the test on each fetus. The ability to test each fetus is affected by the position of each baby in the uterus.

The Biophysical Profile

- A biophysical profile is an in-depth test to examine the babies during the last 2 months of pregnancy.
- It helps determine fetal health and is done when there is need for reassurance about the babies or when there is concern about fetal well-being. The test evaluates the well-being of your babies inside your uterus.
- The test is usually done in high-risk situations, overdue pregnancies or pregnancies in which a baby doesn't move very much.
- It's also useful in evaluating intrauterine-growth restriction.
- A biophysical profile uses a particular scoring system. The first four of the five tests listed in this discussion are made with ultrasound; the fifth is done with external fetal monitors.
- A biophysical profile is a nonstress test combined with ultrasound evaluations.

The Good, the Bad and the Snuggly

"I was only carrying twins, but at 29 weeks my OB-GYN told me my uterus was the size of someone at 40 weeks, carrying one baby, ready to deliver. My babies were 6 weeks early, and they were still 4 pounds and 5 pounds. I have no idea what they would have weighed had I carried them to full term!" —*Betsy*

- A score is given to each of the five areas of evaluation, which include:
  - ~ fetal breathing movements—even though a baby doesn't actually breathe air, the chest wall does move in and out
  - ~ fetal body movements
  - ~ fetal tone
  - ~ amount of amniotic fluid
  - ~ reactive fetal heart rate (nonstress test)
- Fetal "breathing" involves the movement or expansion of a baby's chest inside the uterus. This score is based on the amount of fetal breathing that occurs.
- The baby's body movements are noted. A normal score indicates normal body movements. An abnormal score is given when there are few or no body movements during the allotted time period.
- Fetal tone evaluation is similar and involves rating the movement, or lack of movement, of the baby's arms and legs.

- Evaluating the amount of amniotic fluid requires experience in ultrasound examination. An abnormal test result indicates there is little or no amniotic fluid.
- Fetal heart-rate monitoring (nonstress test) is done with external monitors. It evaluates changes in the fetal heart rate associated with a baby's movements. Evaluations of the amount of change and number of changes in the fetal heart rate differ, depending on who is doing the test and their definition of normal.
- Evaluations may also vary depending on the sophistication of the equipment used and the expertise of the person doing the test.
- For each test, a normal score is 2; an abnormal score is 0. A score of 1 in any of the tests is a middle score.
- From these five scores, a total score is obtained by adding all the values together.
- The higher the score, the better a baby's condition. A lower score may cause concern about the wellbeing of the fetuses.
- A score of 8 to 10 is reassuring; 4 or less is not reassuring.
- If the score is low, your doctor may recommend delivering the babies.
- If the score is reassuring, the test may be repeated at a later date.

- If results fall in the middle, the test may be repeated the following day, depending on the circumstances of the pregnancy and the findings of the biophysical profile.
- The test takes 30 to 40 minutes.
- Your doctor will evaluate all the information before making any decision.

Home Uterine Monitoring

- Some women are monitored at home during pregnancy with home uterine monitoring.
- Contractions of a pregnant woman's uterus are recorded once or more during the day, then transmitted by telephone to the doctor or a nurse for evaluation.
- The procedure is used to monitor women at risk of premature labor.
- Costs vary but run between $80 and $100 a day.

Take Care of Yourself during Pregnancy

One of the most important things to remember with a multiple pregnancy is to take care of yourself from the beginning of your pregnancy until delivery. It's the best way to take care of your developing babies.

- It's important to get adequate rest during pregnancy. This may be difficult because you are getting bigger so fast, but rest when you can. It's harder to carry around two or more babies in your uterus.

- Avoid standing for long periods. This can put a lot of stress on your back and uterus. It can also stress your legs, ankles and feet.

- When you're expecting more than one baby, your nutrition and weight gain are extremely important during pregnancy.

- Food is your best source of nutrients and calories, but it's also important for you to take your prenatal vitamin every day. See the discussion of nutrition, *When You're Eating for More than Two,* that begins on page 73.

- A multiple pregnancy can be more stressful for your body than a single pregnancy, and your needs increase in many areas.

- Often women pregnant with more than one baby have iron-deficiency anemia. See the discussion of *Iron-Deficiency Anemia* that begins on page 29. Iron supplementation is often necessary.

- You may need bed rest as early as your second trimester, or even hospitalization, if you experience complications.
- Bed rest at home or in the hospital can help prevent or stop premature labor. It gives the babies the best chance to grow because bed rest increases blood flow to the uterus. See the discussion of *Bed Rest* that begins on page 70.
- With some multiple pregnancies, planned hospitalization at 28 to 30 weeks may be recommended.

Coping with Discomfort

- When you are expecting more than one baby, your discomfort may be more pronounced; you may experience more problems, or problems may appear sooner and last longer.
- When you are carrying twins, you get "big" earlier, and you are larger than with a single pregnancy. This can cause you more problems, such as difficulty breathing, back pain, hemorrhoids, varicose veins, pelvic pressure and pelvic pain.
- Treatment is often the same for you as for a woman with a singleton pregnancy. Ask your doctor for advice.

Nausea and Vomiting

- You may have to deal with nausea and vomiting during pregnancy; it is also called *morning sickness.*
- Not every woman has morning sickness, but many women do suffer from it.
- Carrying more than one baby may cause morning sickness to be more severe.
- The hormone that makes a home pregnancy test change color—HCG (human chorionic gonado-tropin)—also causes morning sickness.
- The condition usually begins around week 6 and lasts until week 12 or 13, when it starts to taper off.
- Sometimes morning sickness can last all through pregnancy.
- Morning sickness can cause you to avoid food and/or drink, to lose weight and to miss work.
- If you are nauseated, try to keep drinking fluids, even if you can't eat.
- Your body needs lots of fluids all during pregnancy, especially if you lose fluids when you vomit.
- Let your boss know you have morning sickness and that you may miss work sometimes.
- If you normally cook meals, you may want to ask your partner to do it for a while. Your sense of smell may be extra sensitive, which can make you feel sick.

- Acupressure, acupuncture, massage and hypnosis may help you deal with nausea and vomiting.
- Don't take herbs, over-the-counter treatments or any other "remedies" for nausea that are not known to be safe during pregnancy.
- A pill, available by prescription, may help relieve the symptoms of morning sickness; it is called *Bendectin*. Ask your doctor about it if you are interested.

A Severe Problem
- A severe form of morning sickness is called *hyperemesis gravidarum*.
- With hyperemesis gravidarum, a woman has severe nausea, dehydration and vomiting during pregnancy.
- A woman with hyperemesis gravidarum may need to be admitted to the hospital, usually to receive I.V.s to help with dehydration and to receive injectable medications for nausea.
- Hypnosis and/or acupuncture have also been used to help a woman deal with the problem.

Exercising with a Multiple Pregnancy

- As a general rule, women carrying more than one baby are advised *not* to exercise during pregnancy

The Good, the Bad and the Snuggly

"Twins run in my family, on my mother's side. Every generation has a couple of sets, so I wasn't too surprised when the doctor did an ultrasound and told me I was expecting two babies. It was important to be able to talk to my aunts and great aunts about what it was like to have two babies. I got a lot of great information from them—I use it every day!" —*Megan*

because of the extra stress their bodies must deal with and the concern about premature labor and delivery.

- Walking and swimming may be permissible for you for a time, but check with your doctor first.
- If you do get the OK to exercise, don't do anything strenuous—stop immediately if you feel overexerted or if you have any contractions!
- As much as you want to stay in shape, you may have to forgo all exercise programs until after your babies are safely delivered.

Bed Rest

Bed rest is ordered for many women expecting multiples to improve their chances of giving birth to healthy babies. If a woman's condition is severe, hospitalization may be advised.

- When you must rest in bed, it can disrupt normal family routines, especially when bed rest lasts longer than a short time. Adjusting to around-the-clock bed rest can be difficult.
- You may be advised to rest in bed when you are expecting more than one baby. Bed rest may also be advised with the following conditions:
  - ~ a history of premature labor
  - ~ early rupture of the membranes
  - ~ pre-eclampsia
  - ~ high blood pressure
  - ~ premature labor
  - ~ intrauterine-growth restriction
  - ~ diabetes, with complications
- Resting in bed works two ways. First, resting on your side maximizes the blood flow to your uterus, which brings more oxygen and nutrients to the baby. Second, lying down takes the pressure of the babies' weight off the cervix, which can help when a woman experiences premature labor.
- Bed rest can seriously disrupt your routine. You may not be able to work, and you may have to curtail other activities.
- Bed rest can be difficult when you have young children. Changing your routine can be stressful for people around you, including family members and

co-workers. Staying in bed may be hard, but it is better to do it at home than in the hospital!

- Be sure to clarify with your doctor what you can and cannot do while you are on bed rest.

- Sometimes you aren't allowed to get out of bed except to eat, go to the bathroom and go to prenatal appointments.

- At other times, bed rest may be less restricted. You may be able to sit up or be a little more active for part of the day. You may have to take medication and limit your activities.

- You may be advised to lie only on your left side to increase blood flow to the uterus. This position relieves pressure on the vena cava and increases blood flow to the legs and uterus.

- You may be allowed to alternate between sides.

- However, you may *not* lie on your back. Lying on your back puts too much pressure from your uterus on the vena cava, which decreases blood flow to the fetuses and increases edema.

- If you must rest in bed, stay positive! No matter how long you have to rest in bed—a few days or weeks— the goal is healthy babies and a healthy mom. You may be upset or feel anxious, but keep in mind that you're doing this for you and your babies. Give yourself (and everyone else in your family—especially your partner!) a pat on the back.

When You're Eating for More than Two

If you're expecting more than one baby, your nutrition and weight gain are extremely important during your pregnancy. See the discussion of *Target Weight Gain with Multiples* on page 37. It's probably a subject you want to discuss with your doctor as soon as you learn you're going to have more than one baby. He or she may suggest you see a nutritionist.

- When a woman is expecting multiples, there's a bigger nutritional drain on her system.
- If you don't gain weight early in pregnancy, you have a greater chance of developing pre-eclampsia. Your babies may also be tiny.
- If you're expecting twins, target weight gain (for a normal-weight woman) is between 35 and 45 pounds.
- Don't be alarmed when your doctor discusses the amount of weight he or she wants you to gain. Studies show that if a woman gains the targeted amount of weight with a multiple pregnancy, her babies are often healthier.

- You can meet most of your pregnancy nutrition needs by eating a well-balanced, varied diet.
- The *quality* of your calories is important—if you eat a food in its natural state, it's better for you than if it is processed and comes from a can or a box.
- To help you determine if you are choosing healthy foods, buy a book that lists the nutritional content of foods and beverages. There are many available; check your bookstore.
- Reading labels on various food packages can also tell you a lot. If you haven't done this before, try it. You'll learn a great deal about the foods you eat, and it will help you eat healthfully.

Your Healthy Eating Plan

Eating healthfully will go a long way toward giving your babies a healthy start in life. The foods you eat help your babies develop and grow—your babies get the nutrients they need from your blood by way of the placenta.

- When you are eating for yourself and two or more babies, you face a pretty big challenge.
- How can you gain the amount of weight you need to gain? Just adding extra calories won't benefit you or your developing babies.

What Should I Eat?

You may be wondering what kinds of foods to eat, and how much of each, during pregnancy. The chart below offers you some general guidance.

Foods to Eat	*Minimum Servings per Day*
Dark green or dark yellow fruits and vegetables	1
Vitamin-C fruits and vegetables, such as tomatoes and citrus	2
Other fruits and vegetables	4
Whole-grain breads and cereals	6
Dairy products, including milk	5
Protein sources (meat, poultry, eggs, fish)	3
Dried beans and peas, seeds and nuts	2

Foods to Eat in Moderation	
Caffeine	200mg
Fat	limited amounts
Sugar	limited amounts

Foods to Avoid	
Anything containing alcohol	
Food additives, when possible	

- Junk food, full of empty calories, doesn't add much nutrition to your diet.
- You should eat about 3500 calories a day for twins and 4500 calories a day for triplets.

- Add one more serving each of dairy products and protein each day. (These have been included in the chart on page 75.) These two servings provide the extra calcium, protein and iron necessary for you to help meet the needs of your growing babies.
- Eat frequent, small meals during the day to supply better nutrition to your growing babies. Eating six to eight small meals a day is better for you than eating three large meals.
- If you eat three large meals, nutrient levels rise and fall during the day, which isn't as good for the developing fetuses.
- Eating small meals frequently can also help avoid some problems, such as heartburn and indigestion.
- If you eat six times a day, aim for about 600 calories per meal if you are carrying twins and 750 calories per meal if you're carrying triplets.
- Good food choices can provide you with the necessary amounts of protein, calories and calcium. Food is your best source of nutrients and calories, but it's also important for you to take your prenatal vitamin every day.
- Taking a daily prenatal vitamin provides some assurance that you are getting some of the nutrients you need.

The Good, the Bad and the Snuggly

"When I went to the doctor after I found out I was having triplets, I was blown away by the amount of weight she told me I'd have to gain—up to 60 pounds! I said, 'No way,' but she explained to me how *not* gaining the weight could actually harm my babies. I didn't gain the entire 60 pounds, but I was close. She told me after my two girls and one boy were born they were probably healthier because I had paid attention to my nutrition and gained enough weight. And I'm pleased to say that after 2 years, nearly all of my 'baby weight' is gone." —*Tricia*

- In addition, dietary supplements can help you a great deal. See the discussion of *Vitamins and Minerals* beginning on page 88.
- Plan your food intake carefully. Eat proteins and carbohydrates together to help stabilize your blood sugar.
- A serving from the dairy group before bed is a good idea. It helps keep your blood sugar level during the night because it is metabolized slowly.
- For women who need extra help during pregnancy, supplements are often prescribed, especially if you are expecting more than one baby.
- Additional folate may be necessary for a multiple pregnancy.

Food-Group Recommendations

- To get the nutrition you need during your pregnancy, make good food choices.
- Eat the recommended number of servings from each food group every day.
- Eating the right foods, in the correct amounts, takes planning.
- It may help to realize that some foods contain more than one nutrient. For example, yogurt and cheese each provide calcium and protein. One food fills two requirements!
- Choose foods high in vitamins and minerals, especially iron, calcium, magnesium, folic acid and zinc. We give you some food choices for these vitamins and minerals in later discussions.
- You need to eat vitamin-rich foods. Don't expect your prenatal vitamin to provide all the minerals and vitamins you and your babies need—it's *not* a substitute for food.
- Always read food labels—they contain lots of different types of information. Labels help you see what foods are good for you and which ones you should avoid or eat only once in awhile.
- If you have questions or concerns, discuss your nutrition plan with your doctor or a registered dietitian.

Where You Can Find the Nutrients You Need

This chart shows you where to get the various nutrients that you should be eating every day during your pregnancy. We discuss each food group below to help you make good food choices.

Nutrient (Daily Requirement)	Food Sources
Calcium (3000mg; 3g)	Dairy products, dark leafy vegetables, dried beans and peas, tofu, sardines, fortified whole-grain products
Folic acid (0.4mg)	Liver, dried beans and peas, eggs, broccoli, whole-grain products, oranges, orange juice, dark leafy vegetables, legumes, nuts, fortified whole-grain products
Iron (30mg)	Fish, liver, lean red meat, poultry, egg yolks, nuts, dried beans and peas, dark leafy vegetables, dried fruit, fortified whole-grain products
Magnesium (320mg)	Dried beans and peas, cocoa, fish, fortified whole-grain products, nuts, dark leafy vegetables
Vitamin A (770mcg)	Carrots, dark leafy vegetables, sweet potatoes
Vitamin B_6 (2.2mg)	Whole-grain products, liver, meat, bananas, nuts, dried beans, legumes
Vitamin C (85mg)	Citrus, broccoli, tomatoes
Vitamin E (10mg)	Milk, eggs, meats, fish, cereals, dark leafy vegetables, vegetable oils, fortified whole-grain products, nuts, dried beans, legumes
Zinc (15mg)	Fish, meat, nuts, milk, dried beans and peas

Dairy Products

- You need at least 5 servings every day of various dairy products.
- These products contain calcium, which is important for you and your growing babies.
- Foods you might choose from this group, and their serving sizes, include:
  - ~ ¾ cup cottage cheese
  - ~ 2 ounces processed cheese (such as American cheese)
  - ~ 1 ounce hard cheese (such as Parmesan or Romano)
  - ~ 1 cup pudding or custard
  - ~ 1 8-ounce glass of milk (whole, 2%, 1%, skim)
  - ~ 1½ ounces natural cheese (such as cheddar)
  - ~ 1 cup yogurt

Protein Sources

- Pregnancy increases your protein needs.
- Protein is very important to the healthy development of your babies because it contains amino acids.
- Amino acids are critical to the growth and repair of the embryo/fetus, placenta, uterus and breasts.

- You need about 9 to 12 ounces of protein every day; this is more than twice the amount recommended for women who are not pregnant.
- Foods you might choose from the protein group, and their serving sizes, include:
  - ~ 2 tablespoons peanut butter
  - ~ ½ to 1 cup cooked dried beans (check out each one)
  - ~ 2 to 4 ounces cooked meat
  - ~ 1 egg
  - ~ 1 ounce cheese
  - ~ 1 ounce nuts
  - ~ 8 ounces milk
  - ~ 1 ounce tuna, packed in water (limit yourself to 6 ounces of canned tuna a week; see the discussion of *Facts about Fish* on page 84)
  - ~ 8 ounces yogurt

Fruits and Vegetables

- Fruits and vegetables are important in your nutrition plan because they are excellent sources of vitamins, minerals and fiber.
- You need 4 servings of vegetables and at least 3 servings of fruit each day.

- Eating a variety of these foods supplies you with iron, folic acid, calcium, fiber and vitamin C.
- Eat at least one leafy, green or deep-yellow vegetable a day for extra iron, fiber and folic acid.
- Include 2 servings each day of a fruit rich in vitamin C, such as grapefruit juice or orange slices.
- Have fresh fruits when possible; they are a good source of fiber, which can help relieve symptoms of constipation. Drink 100% juice instead of "fruit drinks."
- Fruits and vegetables you may choose from, and their serving sizes, include:
  - ~ ¾ cup vegetable juice
  - ~ ½ cup broccoli, carrots or other vegetable, cooked or raw
  - ~ 1 medium baked potato
  - ~ 1 cup raw, leafy vegetables (greens)
  - ~ ¾ cup grapes
  - ~ ½ cup fruit juice
  - ~ 1 medium banana, orange or apple
  - ~ ¼ cup dried fruit
  - ~ ¼ cup canned or cooked fruit

Breads, Cereal, Pasta and Rice

- Carbohydrate foods provide the primary source of energy for your developing babies.

- These foods also ensure that your body uses protein efficiently.
- You need at least 6 servings from the carbohydrate group each day. Try to eat more.
- Complex carbohydrates, such as whole-wheat breads, pastas and cereals, can be high in fiber. These are good choices because they provide your body with a constant source of energy and help you feel full longer.
- Check out what a serving size is for carbohydrates. It's easy to get more than one serving in a portion.
- Foods you might choose from this group, and their serving sizes, include:
  - ~ 1 10″ tortilla, corn or flour
  - ~ ½ cup cooked pasta, cereal or rice
  - ~ 1 ounce ready-to-eat cereal
  - ~ ½ medium bagel
  - ~ 1 slice bread
  - ~ 1 medium roll

Fats and Sweets

- Be careful with fats and sweets. Foods in this group are often high in calories but low in nutritional value.
- The total fat you consume *also* includes fats in the foods you eat, such as peanut butter, meats, milk, cheese and other foods you choose.

- Be careful with your intake of butter, margarine, oils, salad dressing, nuts, chocolate and sweets.
- Foods from this group, and their serving sizes, include:
  - ~ 1 tablespoon sugar or honey
  - ~ 1 tablespoon olive oil or other type of oil
  - ~ 1 pat of margarine or butter
  - ~ 1 tablespoon jelly or jam
  - ~ 1 tablespoon prepared salad dressing

Facts about Fish

- Eating fish is healthy; it's particularly good for you during pregnancy.
- **Experts recommend that a pregnant woman eat no more than a total of 12 *ounces* of cooked fish a week;** a typical fish serving is 3 to 6 ounces.
- Many fish choices are an excellent, healthful addition to your diet. They are safe to eat; you can eat them as often as you like, as long as you don't exceed 12 ounces a week.
- Fish contains omega-3 fatty acids. Studies show that during pregnancy, omega-3 fatty acids may help prevent high blood pressure, pre-eclampsia and premature labor.
- Studies have shown that fish oil is important to fetal brain development. One study showed that when a

pregnant woman eats fish oil, it reaches the baby's brain. However, studies show it's best not to take in more than 2.4g of omega-3 fatty acids a day.

- Research shows that women who eat a variety of fish during pregnancy have longer pregnancies and give birth to babies that weigh more. Eating fish may also help lower the risk of premature labor.

- Most fish is low in fat and high in vitamin B, iron, zinc, selenium and copper.

- Some fish should be avoided. See discussion later in this section.

- The list below contains acceptable types of fish and shellfish to choose from. If you need to watch your calories, have your choices baked, broiled or steamed. Avoid lots of butter and deep frying.

bass (not large-mouth or sea bass)	ocean perch
	orange roughy
catfish, farm-raised	oysters (not Gulf Coast)
clams	Pacific halibut
crab	perch, freshwater
croaker	red snapper
fish sticks	salmon
flounder	scallops
haddock	scrod
herring	shrimp
lobster	sole
mackerel	trout, farm-raised

The Good, the Bad and the Snuggly

"Having to leave my twins in the hospital while I went home was one of the hardest things I have ever done. I was really depressed when we drove out of the parking lot without them. But they needed to stay there to get healthy enough to come home. One of my babies was a lot sicker than the other one, so he stayed longer. It was a difficult time for all of us, but it was a day of celebration when we were finally all home together!" —*Carrie*

- The FDA recommends removing the skin and as much fat as possible before you eat any type of fish.
- We advise pregnant women not to eat sushi; however, there are a couple of sushi dishes that are OK to eat. Sushi made with *cooked* eel and rolls with *steamed* crab and veggies are acceptable.
- Pregnant women and nursing moms should not eat some types of fish because they are contaminated with a dangerous substance as the result of man-made pollution. People who eat these fish are at risk of methyl-mercury poisoning.
- We know methyl mercury can pass from mother to fetus across the placenta.
- Because of rapid brain development, a fetus may be more vulnerable to methyl-mercury poisoning.
- Other environmental pollutants can appear in fish. Dioxin and PCBs (polychlorinated biphenyls) are

found in some fish, such as bluefish or lake trout; avoid them.

- Parasites, bacteria, viruses and toxins can also contaminate fish. Raw shellfish, if contaminated, could cause hepatitis-A, cholera or gastroenteritis.
- **Avoid all raw fish during pregnancy!**
- **Do not eat** bluefish, Gulf Coast oysters, halibut, king mackerel, lake trout, large-mouth bass, marlin, pike, sea bass, shark, swordfish, tilefish, tuna steaks or tuna sushi, walleye or white croaker during your pregnancy.
- **Avoid some fish** found in warm tropical waters, especially Florida, the Caribbean and Hawaii. Don't eat the following "local" fish from those areas—amberjack, barracuda, grouper, mahimahi and snapper.
- Some freshwater fish may also be risky to eat. To be on the safe side, consult local or state authorities for any advisories on eating freshwater fish.
- Some kinds of fish should not be eaten more than once a month. These fish include blue mussels, cod, eastern oysters, Great Lakes salmon, Gulf of Mexico blue crab, lake whitefish, pollock and wild channel catfish.
- If you are unsure about whether you should eat a particular fish or if you would like further information,

call the Food and Drug Administration on its toll-free telephone hotline: 800-332-4010.

Vitamins and Minerals

- Pregnancy increases your need for vitamins and minerals—a multiple pregnancy increases these needs even more. Vitamins and minerals are an important part of your good nutrition.
- Eating a nutritious variety of food helps you get all the vitamins and minerals you need. It's probably best if you can meet most of these needs through the foods you eat, but this may be difficult for some women.
- That's one reason your doctor prescribes a prenatal vitamin for you—to help meet increased pregnancy needs.
- For women who need extra help during pregnancy, supplements are often prescribed. Your doctor will talk to you about vitamins and minerals, if he or she believes you may need them. If you need more than a prenatal vitamin, he or she will advise you.
- *Caution:* Never take any supplements without your doctor's knowledge, approval and consent!

Getting Enough Calcium

- Calcium is important in the diet of every woman. The daily requirement for a nonpregnant woman is between 800 and 1000mg of calcium.
- When you're pregnant, your needs increase because your growing babies need calcium to build strong bones and teeth, and you need calcium to keep your bones healthy.
- During a singleton pregnancy, your needs increase to 1200mg a day. When you carry more than one baby, your needs increase even more. Ask your doctor how much calcium you should be taking with a multiple pregnancy. Some experts recommend 3g a day with a multiple pregnancy.
- If you don't get enough calcium, your babies may draw needed calcium from your bones, which increases your risk of developing osteoporosis later in life.
- Your body cannot process more than 500mg of calcium at one time, so don't eat all your calcium foods at the same time.
- Extra calcium may help reduce the risk of pre-eclampsia.
- Most prenatal vitamins contain only a portion of the calcium you need.

- Dairy products are great sources of calcium and vitamin D, which is necessary for calcium absorption. It may be difficult for you to get enough calcium without eating dairy foods.
- Various foods are now calcium fortified, such as some orange juice and some breads.
- If dairy products don't appeal to you, add calcium to your diet with fortified juices, tofu and soy milk with added calcium. Other nondairy foods that contain calcium include broccoli, bok choy, collards, kale, mustard greens, spinach, salmon, sardines, garbanzo beans (chickpeas), sesame seeds, almonds, dried beans and trout.
- Some foods interfere with your body's absorption of calcium. Be very careful about consuming salt, protein, tea, coffee and unleavened bread with a calcium-containing food.
- If you and your doctor decide calcium supplements are necessary, you will probably be advised to take calcium carbonate combined with magnesium, which aids calcium absorption.

Your Folic-Acid Intake

- Folic acid (a term used interchangeably with *folate* and vitamin B_9) is a B vitamin that can contribute to a healthy pregnancy.

The Good, the Bad and the Snuggly

"I'm Asian, and there has never been a set of twins in my family, so everyone was really excited when they learned we were having two babies. My mother and mother-in-law waited on me hand and foot while I was pregnant. And when the babies were born, we had relatives and friends standing in line to help out. Everyone wanted to take care of the babies. All the assistance and attention was wonderful, and it helped me get back on my feet very quickly." —*May Ling*

- Folic acid is not stored in the body for very long, so it must be replaced every day.
- A pregnant woman's body excretes four or five times the normal amount of folic acid.
- Some women may need folic acid in addition to that found in prenatal vitamins.
- Deficiency in folic acid can result in a type of anemia called *megaloblastic anemia.*
- Additional folate may be necessary for a pregnancy with twins or triplets because folic-acid requirements are very high.
- In 1998, the U.S. government ordered that some grain products, including flour, breakfast cereals and pasta, be fortified with folic acid.
- Folic acid is also found in many other foods, including bananas, black beans, broccoli, egg yolks, fortified

breads and cereals, green beans, leafy green vegetables, lentils, liver, oranges and other citrus fruits and juices, peas, plantains, spinach, strawberries, tuna, wheat germ and yogurt.

Your Iron Intake

- Iron is one of the most important elements for your body; women need more iron than men because of menstruation.
- The average woman's diet seldom contains enough iron to meet the increased demands of pregnancy (30mg/day). With a multiple pregnancy, that need is even greater.
- Iron needs increase during pregnancy because your blood volume increases by 50% to support the oxygen needs of your babies and the placenta(s).
- Prenatal vitamins contain about 60mg of iron.
- If you have an iron deficiency, you may feel tired, have trouble concentrating, get sick easily or suffer from headaches, dizziness or indigestion.
- An easy way to check for iron deficiency is to examine the inside of your bottom eyelid—it should be dark pink. Or look at your nail beds; if you're getting enough iron, they will be pink.
- The best type of iron to take in is "heme" iron, which comes from sources that contain blood, such

as meat, poultry, eggs and fish. With iron that is not heme-based, the absorption rate is only about 10% and is affected by everything you eat.

- The iron in supplements is *not* heme-based.
- Instead of taking iron supplements, you might want to try to take in heme iron to meet your iron needs.
- In the third trimester, your need for iron increases even more. Your babies draw on your stores to create their own stores for the first few months of life.
- You will also need adequate iron reserves to draw on after the birth because you will lose some blood during delivery.
- To ensure you have enough iron in your diet, eat a lot of iron-rich foods. These include chicken, lean red meat, dried fruits, egg yolks, spinach, kale, tofu and organ meats, such as liver, heart and kidneys.
- Your body stores iron efficiently, so you don't need to eat these foods every day. However, you do need to eat them on a regular basis.
- Eat vitamin-C foods and iron-rich foods together because iron is more easily absorbed by the body when consumed with vitamin C. (A spinach salad with orange sections is a nutritious example.)
- You may not need extra iron if you eat a healthful diet and take your prenatal vitamins every day. Talk to your doctor about it.

- Iron supplements can cause constipation. Work with your doctor to minimize this side effect while making sure you get enough of this important mineral.
- Don't drink tea or coffee with iron-rich foods because tannins present in those beverages inhibit iron absorption by 75%.
- Don't take calcium and iron supplements at the same time, for better absorption of both.

Zinc

- Zinc stabilizes the genetic code in cells and ensures normal tissue growth in the fetuses. You need about 15mg each day.
- This mineral helps prevent miscarriage and premature delivery and can help regulate blood sugar in you and your babies.
- Zinc also plays a critical role in immune functions; it helps fight infection.
- It may also help your babies gain weight.
- In addition, zinc may help prevent stretch marks, which can be more of a problem with a multiple pregnancy.
- Prenatal vitamins include 15 to 25mg of zinc, an adequate amount for most women. Ask your doctor if you need more than this amount.

- This mineral is found in many foods, including seafood, meat, nuts and milk.
- Lima beans, whole-grain products, dried beans and peas, wheat germ and dark leafy vegetables are all good nonmeat sources of this mineral.

Vitamin A
- Vitamin A is essential to human reproduction.
- Deficiency of vitamin A in North America is rare; most women have adequate stores of the vitamin in the liver.
- What concerns doctors now is the *excessive use* of vitamin A before conception and during early pregnancy. (This concern extends only to vitamin A derived from fish oils. Vitamin A from plants is believed to be safe.)
- Studies indicate that high levels during pregnancy of vitamin A from fish oil may cause birth defects, including cleft palate and "water on the brain" (hydrocephalus).
- The recommended daily allowance (RDA) of vitamin A is 2700IU (international units) a day for a woman of childbearing age (5000IU is a maximum dosage).
- The requirement is the same for pregnant and nonpregnant women.

- Most women get the vitamin A they need during pregnancy from the foods they eat.
- Supplementation during pregnancy is not recommended.
- Be cautious about taking *any* substances that you have not discussed with your doctor, including vitamin A.
- If you have questions, ask your physician.

Vitamin B

- The B vitamins—B_6, B_{12} and folic acid (B_9)—influence fetal development of nerves and red blood cells.
- Nearly 40% of all Americans are close to a deficiency in vitamin B_{12}.
- If your vitamin-B_{12} level is low, you could develop anemia during pregnancy.
- Milk, eggs, tempeh and miso provide vitamins B_6 and B_{12}. Other good sources of B_6 include bananas, potatoes, collard greens, avocados and brown rice.

Vitamin E

- Vitamin E is important during pregnancy because it helps metabolize fats and helps build fetal muscles and red blood cells. You need about 10mg of vitamin E a day.

- You can usually get enough of this vitamin if you eat meat.
- If you don't eat meat, it can be harder to get vitamin E from the rest of your diet.
- Unbleached, cold-pressed vegetable oils (such as olive oil), wheat germ, spinach and dried fruits are all good sources of vitamin E.
- Read the label on your prenatal vitamin, or ask your doctor if your prenatal vitamin contains 100% of the RDA for vitamin E.

Other Supplements
- The benefit of *fluoride supplementation* during pregnancy is controversial. Some prenatal vitamins contain fluoride.
- Some researchers believe fluoride supplementation in a pregnant woman results in improved teeth in her child, but not everyone agrees.
- Fluoride supplementation during pregnancy has not been found to harm a baby.
- You might want to talk to your doctor about taking extra *magnesium.*
- Magnesium helps to relax muscles; the uterus is a muscle.
- It might help reduce preterm labor if you take magnesium throughout your pregnancy. Ask your doctor about it.

The Good, the Bad and the Snuggly

"I had had three children before I got pregnant with my twins. I felt I was an old hand at the mother game. However, I was in for a shock when my daughters were born. It was a lot harder to take care of two babies at once—one was very ill, even after we brought her home from the hospital. And my three other kids needed me. I hired a nurse to come in each night for the first 8 weeks. That helped me get some much-needed rest and allowed me to spend some quality time with my three 'big kids.'" —*Kim*

Your Prenatal Vitamin Is Important

- Did the doctor prescribe prenatal vitamins for you to take during pregnancy? If not, you should bring this up at your next office visit.
- Most pregnant women take a daily prenatal vitamin to meet the increased demands on their bodies for more vitamins and minerals while their babies are growing and developing.
- Each prenatal vitamin contains many essential ingredients for the development of your babies and for your good health.
- You should take one *every day* until your babies are born.
- A typical prenatal vitamin contains:

- ~ calcium to build your babies' teeth and bones, and to help strengthen your own
- ~ copper to help prevent anemia and to help bone formation
- ~ folic acid to reduce the risk of neural-tube defects and to help blood-cell production
- ~ iodine to help control metabolism
- ~ iron to prevent anemia, and to help your babies' blood development
- ~ vitamin A for general health and body metabolism
- ~ vitamin B_1 for general health and body metabolism
- ~ vitamin B_2 for general health and body metabolism
- ~ vitamin B_3 for general health and body metabolism
- ~ vitamin B_6 for general health and body metabolism
- ~ vitamin B_{12} to promote formation of blood
- ~ vitamin C to aid your body's absorption of iron
- ~ vitamin D to strengthen your babies' bones and teeth, and to help your body use phosphorus and calcium
- ~ vitamin E for general health and body metabolism
- ~ zinc to help balance fluids in your body and to aid nerve and muscle function
- If you are ill, such as with the flu, and cannot keep food or liquid down, don't take your prenatal vitamin. Begin taking it again when you feel better.

Drink Enough Fluid

- Water is essential to a healthy pregnancy. It enables your body to process nutrients, develop new cells, keep up with blood-volume increases and regulate body temperature.
- Your blood volume increases during pregnancy; drinking extra fluids helps you keep up with this change.
- Research has shown that for every 15 calories you burn, your body needs about 1 tablespoon of water. If you burn 2000 calories a day, you need 133 tablespoons—2 quarts—of water!
- Because you need more calories during pregnancy, you also need more water.
- Drink eight 8-ounce glasses (2 quarts) or more of liquid every day.
- Many pregnant women who suffer from headaches, uterine cramping and other problems find that if they increase their water or fluid intake, some symptoms are relieved.
- In addition, extra fluid may provide other benefits, including boosting endurance and easing constipation.
- Drinking plenty of water also helps avoid bladder infections.

- To determine if you're drinking enough fluid, check your urine. When it is light yellow to clear, you're getting enough water. Dark-yellow urine is a sign you need to increase your fluid intake.

Meal Plans

During pregnancy, you need high quality nutrition, but it should taste good, too! The menus listed below supply you with the nutrition you need to help you give your babies the nutrients they need to grow and to develop. These meal plans are for a woman carrying twins; they include the extra calories you need and additional dairy and protein servings.

DAY 1
Breakfast
    2 waffles
    1 T syrup
    2 strips of bacon
    1 cup milk
    ¾ cup mixed fruit
Snack
    1 English muffin
    2 T jam
    3 ounces of hard cheese

Lunch

    2 slices multigrain bread

    4 ounces cooked chicken breast

    1 T mayonnaise

    ½ cup cottage cheese

    tomato-and-lettuce salad

    1 cup milk

Snack

    10 whole-wheat crackers

    ¼ cup hummus

    1 carton flavored yogurt

Dinner

    1 4-ounce pork chop, fat removed

    1 cup cooked pasta

    1 T margarine for pasta

    sliced tomatoes and mozarella cheese

    1 small roll

    1 glass water with lemon

Snack

    ½ cup pudding

    4 vanilla wafers

    1 cup hot chocolate

DAY 2

Breakfast

    1 fruit-and-yogurt smoothie

    1 medium banana-nut muffin

    1 medium plum

Snack

    1 cup lowfat cottage cheese

    1 medium orange, cut into chunks

Lunch

   2 cups vegetable soup

   1 whole-wheat roll

   2 ounces cheese

   1 cup milk

Snack

   ½ cup bean dip

   10 saltine crackers

   1 small milkshake

Dinner

   4 ounces beef steak

   1 medium sweet potato

   1 T margarine for potato

   1 cup Caesar salad

   1 cup mixed vegetables

   1 cup milk

Snack

   2 ounces cheddar cheese

   10 crackers

   1 cup cranberry juice

DAY 3

Breakfast

   1 two-egg omelet with cheese

   2 pieces toast

   2 T margarine

   1 cup calcium-fortified grapefruit juice

Snack

   1 medium blueberry muffin

   ½ cup yogurt

   ¼ cup mixed nuts

Lunch

　　2 slices whole-wheat bread
　　½ can tuna, packed in water
　　2 T mayonnaise for sandwich
　　tomato and lettuce for sandwich
　　10 baked potato chips
　　1 cup milk

Snack

　　½ peanut-butter sandwich
　　¼ cup raisins
　　2 small cookies

Dinner

　　4 ounces chicken
　　1 cup pasta salad
　　1 cup green beans
　　sliced tomatoes
　　1 small roll
　　1 cup milk

Snack

　　1 bagel
　　2 T cream cheese
　　1 small yogurt shake

Other Pregnancy Considerations

Working during Pregnancy

Often a physician advises a woman expecting twins to stop working at least 8 weeks before her due date. Ideally, you

The Good, the Bad and the Snuggly

"Being an older pregnant woman was hard enough, but being an older mom with my first children—triplet boys—seemed to increase my needs for rest, exercise and good nutrition. I have always paid attention to my lifestyle, so it wasn't as hard to get into a routine after the babies were born that focused on me a little. I asked my husband, my family and friends to pitch in whenever they could. When they did, I took some time for myself so I could do things that would help me recover and be strong for the wild ride I knew I'd be taking with three boys growing up under one roof!" —*Marie*

should stop working at 28 weeks with a twin pregnancy—24 weeks if your job requires standing or other physical exertion. Your doctor may recommend full or partial bed rest. These are only general suggestions and may not apply in every case. Your doctor will make a recommendation based on your unique situation and work conditions. A woman pregnant with triplets or more may have to begin her leave even earlier.

Childbirth-Education Classes

It's a great idea to take childbirth-education classes for any pregnancy. Begin looking into classes that are offered in your area around 16 weeks of pregnancy. If you're expecting twins, triplets or more, schedule your classes to begin at least *3* to *4 months* before your due date. If you have time, a brief course in Cesarean birth might also be worthwhile, if you can find one in your area.

- Prenatal classes are not only for first-time pregnant women. If you have a new partner, if it has been a few years since you've had a baby, if you have questions or if you would like a review of what lies ahead, a prenatal class can help you.

- These classes may help reduce any worries or concerns you and your partner have about labor and delivery. They can help you enjoy the birth of your babies even more.

- Today, you may even be able to find a childbirth-education class for parents expecting multiples. Ask your doctor about them.

- Most childbirth-education classes run 4 to 6 weeks—you and your labor coach attend one class each week.

- Practice what you learn in your classes. Try to practice for at least 20 minutes a day or as much as the instructor suggests. If you can't practice 20 minutes a day, four 30-minute sessions each week should be beneficial.

- Check out the qualifications of the person teaching the class. Some instructors are medically trained, such as a labor-and-delivery nurse; others have no medical training at all.

- Once you have found a class you think will work for you, find out how long it lasts, how much it costs, what the class curriculum includes, the instructor's credentials and the childbirth philosophy of the class (is there just one, or are different philosophies presented?). Then you and your partner will be able to decide whether a particular class is just right for you!

Premature Birth

Preterm or *premature* birth refers to any birth that occurs more than 3 weeks before the estimated due date. About 10% of all babies are born prematurely.

- Recent statistics show that over 60% of all deliveries of multiples in the United States were preterm (born earlier than 37 weeks). In the past 5 years, this rate has increased nearly 25%.
- The more fetuses in a pregnancy, the greater the chance of premature birth. Over 90% of all triplet births and nearly every birth of higher-number fetuses are premature.

- On average, twin pregnancies deliver around 36 weeks, triplets at 32 weeks, quadruplets at 30 weeks and quintuplets at 29 weeks.
- Studies have shown that 28 weeks seems to be the magical point at which complication rates drop significantly with multiples.
- It's interesting to note that twins born at 37 to 38 weeks fare better as newborns than those born later in pregnancy. A due date of 40 weeks does not seem appropriate for twins!
- Signs of premature labor you may experience include:
  - ~ discharge from the vagina, or an increase in vaginal discharge
  - ~ a change in vaginal discharge; it becomes more watery or bloody
  - ~ feeling pressure in the lower abdominal or pelvic area
  - ~ constant low, dull backache
  - ~ mild abdominal cramps, with or without diarrhea
  - ~ regular contractions or tightening of the uterus
  - ~ your bag of waters breaks
- Premature birth increases the risk of problems in a baby. Babies born prematurely usually weigh less than 5½ pounds. Potential problems in the babies include:
  - ~ low birth weight

- ~ developmental disabilities
- ~ respiratory/lung problems
- ~ cerebral palsy
- Preterm delivery of a baby can be serious because a baby's lungs and other systems may not be ready to function on their own.
- It's usually best for the babies to remain in the uterus as long as possible so they can grow and develop fully.
- Your doctor may take steps to halt contractions if you go into labor too early.
- Follow all instructions from your doctor to help deal with this problem.
- In most cases, the causes of premature labor and premature birth are unknown. Causes we do understand include multiple fetuses, a uterus with an abnormal shape, too much amniotic fluid, placental abruption, placenta previa, vasa previa, premature rupture of membranes, an incompetent cervix, abnormalities of the fetus, fetal death, a retained IUD, serious maternal illness or incorrect estimate of gestational age.
- One test, called *SalEst,* can help determine if a woman might go into labor too early.
- The test measures levels of the hormone estriol in a pregnant woman's saliva. There may be a surge in this chemical several weeks before early labor.

- A positive result means a woman has a 7 times higher chance of delivering her babies before the 37th week of pregnancy.
- Another test your doctor may do is a *fetal fibronectin (fFN) test.*
- There is a lower risk of preterm birth when the test result for fFN is negative after 22 weeks and before 35 weeks of pregnancy. See the discussion of the *Fetal Fibronectin (fFN) Test* on page 56.

Treatment of Premature Labor

- Half of all twins and 9 out of 10 triplets are born prematurely.
- Beginning around week 20 of your pregnancy, your doctor will probably begin monitoring you closely for signs of premature labor. Monitoring may alert your doctor to problems you are having; treatment may be initiated to keep you and your babies safe.
- To help determine whether premature labor is a possibility, your doctor may do an internal exam or recommend a vaginal ultrasound to see if your cervix is shortening (which may indicate labor could start soon).
- Electronic fetal monitoring may also be done.

- If your doctor monitors you and finds you are at risk for premature delivery, different treatment options are available.
- The treatment most often used for premature labor is bed rest.
- Not everyone agrees on this treatment, but bed rest is often successful in stopping contractions and premature labor.
- If you are advised to rest in bed, it may mean you can't go to work or continue many activities.
- It's worth it to agree to bed rest if it will prevent premature delivery of your babies.
- Beta-adrenergic agents, also called *tocolytic agents,* may be used to suppress labor.
- Beta-adrenergics are muscle relaxants. They relax the uterus and decrease contractions. (The uterus is mainly muscle; it is the tightening or contraction of the uterus that pushes a baby out through the cervix during labor.)
- At this time, only *ritodrine (Yutopar)* is approved by the FDA to treat premature labor.
- Ritodrine is approved for use between 20 and 36 weeks of pregnancy.
- Ritodrine is given in three different forms—intravenously, as an intramuscular injection and as a pill.

The Good, the Bad and the Snuggly

"I tried my best to take care of myself when I was pregnant with our triplets. I kept all my doctor's appointments and stayed fairly active taking care of our other three children—boys aged 4, 6 and 7. I had a maternity shirt printed up that I liked to wear. It read, 'Not one, not two, but three . . . and no drugs!' It meant I was carrying triplets, and they were conceived without the help of any fertility drugs. My doctor told me that's pretty rare!" —*Molly*

- In some cases, the medication is used in women with a history of premature labor or for a woman with multiple pregnancies.
- It is initially given intravenously and may require a hospital stay of a couple of days or more.
- When premature contractions stop, you may be switched to oral medications, which you take every 2 to 4 hours.
- *Terbutaline* may also be used as a muscle relaxant to halt premature labor.
- Although it has been shown to be an effective medication and is used frequently for this purpose, it has not been approved for this use by the FDA.
- *Magnesium sulfate* is used to treat pre-eclampsia; we have known for quite a while that magnesium sulfate may also help stop premature labor.

- You must be monitored frequently if you take magnesium sulfate.
- *Sedatives* or *narcotics* may also be used in early attempts to stop labor; this may be an injection of morphine or meperidine (Demerol).
- Use of sedatives or narcotics is not a long-term solution but may be effective in initially stopping labor.
- A recent study showed that use of the hormone *progesterone (17 alpha-hydroxyprogesteronecaproate)* in some women may reduce their risk of giving birth to a premature baby.
- In the study, women who had had problems with premature labor in previous pregnancies were given a weekly injection of progesterone.
- This course of treatment substantially reduced the rate of premature deliveries. More studies are needed, but there is hope that this treatment will lead to a decrease in premature births.
- If you experience premature labor, you may need to see your doctor more frequently.
- Your doctor will probably monitor your pregnancy with ultrasound, nonstress tests, contraction-stress tests and biophysical profiles.
- When premature labor is halted, it reduces the risks of fetal problems and problems related to premature delivery.

- If treatments don't work, and babies will be born before 34 weeks gestation, corticosteroids may be given to you to help speed fetal lung development. This could help reduce the likelihood and/or severity of breathing problems when babies are born.

Delivering More than One Baby

The way multiples are delivered often depends on how the babies are lying in your uterus. Studies show that half of all women carrying twins may be able to have a normal vaginal delivery, if both babies are in the normal head-down position and other conditions are right. It also depends on your babies' weight and health, as well as your health.

- Possible complications of labor and delivery with multiples, in addition to prematurity of the babies, include:
  - ~ abnormal presentations (breech or transverse)
  - ~ prolapse of the umbilical cord(s) (the umbilical cord comes out ahead of a baby)
  - ~ placental abruption
  - ~ fetal stress
  - ~ bleeding after delivery
- Because there is higher risk during labor and delivery, precautions may be taken before delivery and

during labor, including the need for an I.V., the presence of an anesthesiologist and the availability and possible presence of pediatricians or other medical personnel to take care of the babies after birth.

- After delivery of two or more babies, the doctor pays close attention to maternal bleeding because of the rapid change in the size of the uterus. It is greatly overdistended with more than one baby.
- Medication, usually oxytocin (Pitocin), is given by I.V. to cause contractions of the uterus to stop bleeding so the mother doesn't lose too much blood.
- A heavy blood loss could produce anemia and make a blood transfusion or long-term treatment with iron supplementation necessary.

The Babies' Birth Positions

- Most babies enter the birth canal head first (vertex), which is the best presentation for labor and a vaginal delivery.
- With multiples, it becomes complicated because each baby can present differently, and the presentation of the babies still inside the uterus can change after delivery of the preceding baby.

- With twins, when both are head first, a vaginal delivery may be attempted and may be accomplished safely.
- However, it may be possible for only one baby to deliver normally.
- The second one could require a C-section if it turns, if the cord comes out ahead of the baby or if the baby is stressed following delivery of the first fetus.
- Some doctors believe delivery of two or more babies requires a Cesarean delivery.
- There is a difference between birth *presentation* and birth *position.*
- *Presentation* refers to the part of the baby that enters the birth canal first. The terms *breech* and *vertex* refer to presentation, not position.
- *Position* refers to the relation of a part of the baby to the right or left side of the birth canal.
- With twins, there are three main categories of presentations.
    - ~ in 40% of deliveries, both twins are head first (both are vertex)
    - ~ in 40% of deliveries, the first twin is head first (vertex), but the second twin is *not* head first (nonvertex)
    - ~ in 20% of deliveries, the first twin is not head first (nonvertex)

- The possibility of different presentations with triplets and higher numbers is multiplied exponentially.
- A *breech presentation* means the baby is not in a head-down position; its legs or buttocks come into the birth canal first.
- If the first baby is not in the head-down position (vertex), most of the time a doctor will perform a Cesarean delivery.
- The American College of Obstetricians and Gynecologists (ACOG) recommends Cesarean delivery when the first baby is in the breech position. Attempts to turn the first baby have not been very successful.
- One of the main causes of a breech presentation is prematurity of the baby. This is often a consideration with multiples because they are often premature. Many experts believe it is safer to deliver premature babies by Cesarean section, especially if they weigh less than 3 pounds, 5 ounces (1500g).
- Near the end of the second trimester, the babies are commonly in the breech presentation.
- As you move through the third trimester, any of the babies could turn into the head-down or vertex presentation for birth.
- There are other presentations that are not normal.

- A *Frank breech* occurs when a baby's legs are straight and bent at the hips; the baby is in a jack-knife position. Feet are up by the face or head.
- In a *complete breech presentation,* one or both knees are bent.
- With an *incomplete breech presentation,* a foot or knee enters the birth canal ahead of the rest of the baby.
- In a *face presentation,* the baby's head is hyperextended so the face enters the birth canal first.
- If a baby is in a *transverse lie,* it is lying almost as if in a cradle in your pelvis. The head is on one side of your abdomen, and the bottom is on the other side.
- With a *shoulder presentation,* the baby's shoulder enters the birth canal first.
- If you deliver your babies vaginally, it may be necessary to perform an ultrasound after delivery of the first baby to check the presentation of the following baby, or babies. Presentation can change after the birth of the preceding baby. This happens about 20% of the time with twins.
- The hospital where you deliver should have a portable ultrasound machine available in labor and delivery. Discuss this with your doctor if you are considering a vaginal birth.

The Good, the Bad and the Snuggly

"It was hard having three sisters who seemed to get pregnant at the drop of a hat. One or more of them was having a baby every year, while my success at pregnancy was dismal. They had gorgeous little families; I suffered through two miscarriages, one ectopic pregnancy and endless infertility tests and treatments, including surgery. And we still couldn't get pregnant! But that's all in the past, now. With the help of a wonderful team of doctors, nurses and other medical professionals, and using assisted-reproductive technology, we were blessed with twins who will celebrate their first birthday this week. Only someone that has endured what Dave and I have will understand how precious our two girls are to us." —*Dayna*

- The need may arise for an immediate Cesarean delivery of the second baby following the birth of the first. Find out if the hospital you are going to is capable of performing an emergency Cesarean delivery, if one is necessary.

Delivering a Breech Baby

- For many years, most breech deliveries were performed vaginally. Then it was believed the safest method was Cesarean delivery, especially if it was a first baby.

- Many doctors today believe a Cesarean delivery is still the safest method of delivering a breech baby. With multiples, this is especially true if the first baby is breech.
- Special considerations need to be made with the delivery of multiple fetuses. The maturity of the babies and whether you have had a previous Cesarean delivery are important factors.
- Not everyone agrees how premature multiples should be delivered. Some believe a Cesarean delivery is less traumatic and safer for premature infants.
- Most medical experts agree that when a woman is carrying more than two babies, they should be delivered by Cesarean delivery.
- Ask your doctor what he or she normally does in this situation, and ask if the hospital where you plan to deliver can handle emergency Cesarean deliveries.
- *Delayed interval delivery* may occur in a vaginal birth of multiples. This means the first baby is delivered, but the birth of the other baby, or babies, is delayed for a long period of time. The normal interval between births is short, usually less than 30 minutes. With delayed interval delivery, this time period could be hours to days!
- Many problems and dangers can occur with delayed interval delivery, including infection and bleeding

in the mother. In some cases, a cervical cerclage is used to close the cervix.

- Fortunately, delayed interval delivery is a rare occurrence.

Analgesics and Anesthesia

There are many different types of pain relief for labor and delivery. *Analgesia* is pain relief without total loss of sensation. *Anesthesia* is pain relief with partial or total loss of sensation. Analgesia and anesthesia for multiples is complicated by situations related to multiples, such as prematurity, maternal complications, the need for manipulation of the babies during delivery, problems with uterine bleeding or the failure of the uterus to contract after delivery (uterine atony).

Analgesia

- With analgesia, medication is injected into a muscle or vein to decrease the pain of labor; you remain conscious. Examples of medications used for analgesia are Demerol (meperidine) and morphine.
- It provides pain relief but can make you drowsy, restless or nauseous. You may find concentration difficult.

- Analgesia may slow a baby's reflexes and breathing, so this medication is usually given during the early and middle parts of labor so it has time to wear off.

Anesthesia
- There are three types of anesthesia—general anesthesia, local anesthesia and regional anesthesia.
- You are completely unconscious under *general anesthesia,* so it is used only for some Cesarean deliveries and emergency vaginal deliveries.
- With general anesthesia, the babies are also anesthetized and need to be resuscitated after delivery.
- An advantage of general anesthesia is that it can be administered quickly in an emergency.
- *Local anesthesia* affects a small area and is useful for an episiotomy repair.
- It rarely affects the babies and usually has few lingering effects.
- *Regional anesthesia* affects a larger body area. The three most common types of regional anesthesia are epidural blocks, spinal blocks and pudendal blocks.
- Epidural anesthesia is the most commonly used form of pain relief in the United States and provides the most effective pain relief during labor.

- Many doctors prefer epidural anesthesia for multiples, but extra care must be taken to avoid hypotension (low blood pressure) in the mother.
- With an epidural block, a tube is inserted into a space, called the *epidural space,* outside your spinal column in the lower back. Medication is administered through the tube for pain relief, and you remain conscious during labor and delivery.
- An epidural block may be done during labor or for a C-section. It numbs the pain of contractions and can be strong enough to allow a Cesarean delivery to be performed.
- An epidural is usually performed by an anesthesiologist (a medical doctor) or a nurse trained in the procedure (a certified nurse anesthetist, or CNA).
- A spinal block is similar to an epidural; however, it is not usually used in labor but *only* for a C-section or a vaginal delivery. A single dose is given that lasts long enough for a Cesarean delivery to be performed or for a birth, but it doesn't last long enough for labor.
- This type of block is administered only once during labor, so it is often used just before delivery or before the Cesarean section is performed.

- General anesthesia is usually used for emergency Cesarean or vaginal deliveries when there isn't time for an epidural or spinal.
- It is administered using a combination of I.V. and inhaled medications.
- If you receive general anesthesia, you are unconscious or asleep.
- It is critical with the delivery of multiples that skilled anesthetic services are immediately available for either a Cesarean delivery or manipulation of a baby.

Some Risks during Labor

- Failure of the uterus to contract after delivery is a significant risk with multiples.
- Women delivering multiples also have a much higher risk of bleeding during delivery and after the babies' birth (postpartum).
- An important resource to have available at the hospital where you will deliver is blood for a transfusion, if necessary.
- If you are anemic during pregnancy, any bleeding (more than normal) during delivery or after the birth presents a more significant risk than it would for women who are not anemic.

Fetal Monitoring and Testing

- In many hospitals, babies are monitored throughout labor.
- Monitoring with multiples presents some challenges. It means that monitoring of all babies will be continuous during labor.
- With twins, this may be accomplished with an internal monitor on the first baby (membranes must be ruptured and baby must be head first) and an external monitor on the second baby.
- With triplets and more, this can be very difficult. External monitors can be hard to use, especially if the babies move a lot.
- *External fetal monitoring* can be done before your membranes rupture.
- With external monitoring, belts are strapped to your abdomen to record your contractions and the babies' heartbeats.
- One or more straps hold an ultrasound to monitor fetal heart rates. Another strap holds a device to measure the length of contractions and how often they occur.
- *Internal fetal monitoring* monitors a baby more precisely. This type of monitoring can be done on only one baby.

The Good, the Bad and the Snuggly

"*Fetal reduction* sounded like such a cold, clinical term when our infertility specialist mentioned it. Through reading a lot about the subject, I had actually learned the correct term was *multifetal pregnancy reduction*. After all we had been through in the last few years, with the heartbreak of pregnancy loss and difficult infertility tests, the idea of eliminating some of the fetuses that might result from in-vitro fertilization seemed unrealistic to us. However, our doctor explained that if four fetuses 'took' and implanted in my uterus, the best chance of success for any of the babies to make it to delivery might be to eliminate two of them with fetal reduction. Scientifically it made sense, but it still was hard to consider actually doing it. They even told us that tests could be done to check all the fetuses in my uterus to see if they were normal or not, which is called *prenatal genetic diagnosis*. We had some very personal discussions as a couple, and excellent counselors helped us make some difficult decisions." —*Miranda*

- An electrode, called a *scalp electrode,* is placed through the vagina and cervix, then attached to the fetus's scalp to measure the fetal heart rate.
- A thin tube, called an *internal pressure catheter,* can be put inside the uterus to monitor the strength of the contractions.
- This is done *only* after your membranes have ruptured.
- It may be a little uncomfortable to have monitors placed or inserted, but it is not painful.

- Monitors send data to a machine that records the information on a strip of paper.
- Monitor results can usually be seen in your room and at the nurses' station. In some places, your doctor can check results on his or her computer.
- In most cases, you must stay in bed during monitoring. In some places, wireless monitors are available so you can move around.

Monitoring Contractions

- It can be difficult to monitor contractions accurately with multiples.
- Labor with multiples is often complicated by dysfunctional (ineffective) labor; premature separation of the placenta (placental abruption), especially after delivery of the first baby; prolapse of the umbilical cord; cord entanglement; or insufficiency of the placenta (inadequate blood flow to the placenta).
- Care must be taken to see that each baby is monitored, and one baby is not monitored twice.

Evaluating Fetal Lung Maturity

- The respiratory system is the last fetal system to mature.

- Premature infants often have respiratory difficulties because their lungs are not fully developed.
- Knowing how mature the babies' lungs are helps the doctor make a decision about early delivery in cases where that must be considered.
- If the babies need to be delivered early, tests can predict whether they will be able to breathe without assistance.
- There are several fetal lung maturity tests available, including:
  - ~ lecithin/sphingomyelin ratio (L/S ratio)
  - ~ phosphatidyl glycerol (PG)
  - ~ foam stability index
  - ~ fluorescence polarization
  - ~ optical density at 650nm
  - ~ Lamellar body counts
  - ~ saturated phosphatidylcholine
- The test a doctor chooses to use depends on test availability and the experience of those taking care of you in the hospital.
- Two tests used most often to evaluate the babies' lungs before birth are the *L/S ratio* and the *phosphatidyl glycerol (PG)* tests.
- Fluid for these two tests is obtained by amniocentesis.

- With multiples, a decision must be made as to whether fluid will be drawn from around each baby for these determinations.

Test to Determine Babies' Oxygen Levels

- Medical staff can now monitor the babies' oxygen levels *inside* the womb, before birth. Light measures the oxygen level in fetal blood, providing accurate answers as to whether the babies' oxygen levels are in the safe range.
- This test, called *OxiFirst* fetal oxygen monitoring, is used during labor.
- With multiples, only the first baby presenting can be evaluated.
- For this reason, this test is not very helpful with multiples.

Cesarean Delivery of Multiples

- A Cesarean delivery is also called a *C-section.*
- When you have a Cesarean delivery, babies are delivered through an incision made in the mother's abdominal wall and uterus.

- There are many reasons for doing a Cesarean delivery, but the main goal is to deliver healthy babies and to preserve the health of the mother.
- The rate of Cesareans done in the United States is between 20 and 25% of all deliveries.

How a Cesarean Is Performed

- An incision is made through the skin of the lower abdomen down to the uterus, and the wall of the uterus is cut.
- The amniotic sac containing the babies and placenta is cut, and the babies are removed through the incisions. Babies may be in one sac or in individual sacs (the latter is more common).
- After the babies are delivered, the placenta(s) is removed. This is the point at which it should be saved for pathological examination, to determine if babies are monozygotic.
- The uterus is closed in layers with absorbable sutures (they don't have to be removed).
- Finally, the abdomen is sewn together.
- You may have an epidural or spinal anesthetic so you are awake for the procedure. You can see your babies immediately after birth, and your partner can be with you.

- A Cesarean delivery is major surgery and carries with it certain risks, including infection, bleeding, shock through blood loss, the possibility of blood clots and the possibility of injury to other organs, such as the bladder or rectum.
- A Cesarean with multiples may be more difficult than delivery with a single baby.
- With multiples, positioning the woman may be harder because her abdomen is larger; this can cause problems with low blood pressure.
- Often larger incisions are necessary so the babies can be removed safely. This is because the babies can be in many different presentations and positions.
- The uterus often contracts after delivery of the first baby, making it more difficult to remove the remaining baby or babies.
- In addition, because the uterus has been overdistended, it may fail to contract. This can result in heavier bleeding.
- In some multiple births, the first baby delivers vaginally but the second requires a Cesarean delivery. This happens when the second baby changes position, gets tangled in the cord or becomes too stressed to remain in the uterus, or when the placenta separates from the wall of the uterus (placental abruption) after the first baby is born.

- Recovery is slower with a Cesarean than with a vaginal delivery. Full recovery normally takes 4 to 6 weeks. Recovery from a multiple pregnancy could take even longer.

Vaginal Delivery of Multiples

- Most medical authorities agree that delivery of triplets or more should be by Cesarean delivery. Much of this is covered in the discussion of *The Babies' Birth Positions* on page 115.
- As with the birth of any baby, the goal in a multiple delivery is the health of the mother and babies.
- Whether you will attempt to deliver vaginally depends a great deal on the experience and skills of those caring for you.
- The most ideal situation for vaginal delivery of twins is for both babies to be head down. Studies show that about 50% of the time, babies in this situation can be successfully delivered vaginally.
- In most cases, the second baby will deliver within 30 minutes of the first one.
- Emergency situations can occur rapidly; resources such as a portable ultrasound, a blood bank, anesthesia and skilled assistants and nurses are critical.

The Good, the Bad and the Snuggly

"When the TV news reported stories of conjoined or Siamese twins, I usually didn't pay much attention to them. When video was shown, I found it hard to watch and usually turned away or changed the channel. This could never happen to me. But it did. With a previous easy pregnancy, I didn't think I had anything to worry about. About the time we adjusted to the idea of two babies at once, we were shocked when follow-up ultrasound exams showed my unborn daughters were joined at the head. Our pregnancy took on a very serious, scary dimension. Following a lot of planning and a Cesarean delivery, the girls were delivered. Now they are 2 years old, and I sit in the waiting room as they are in surgery. The surgeons are optimistic of a good result. It has been a difficult time, but our family loves the girls more than I could have thought possible." —*Celeste*

- Vaginal birth of multiples should be attempted in hospitals where resources are readily available for an emergency Cesarean delivery and where other complications can be managed.

After Your Babies' Birth

Recovery after the birth of twins, triplets or more may be a little more difficult for several reasons. Your pregnancy may have been harder on your body than a singleton

pregnancy might be. The risk of problems or complications is higher with a multiple pregnancy. You may have
gained more weight or experienced more edema. You
may have had a Cesarean delivery. And you have more
babies to care for.

- A multiple pregnancy often delivers early, so you may
  not have had time to prepare to bring your babies
  home. Gestation for a singleton pregnancy is about
  280 days. For twins, gestation is about 260 days, and
  for triplets, it is about 247 days. This is counting from
  the first day of your last menstrual period.

- Another problem with early delivery is prematurity
  of the babies. If your babies are premature and have
  to stay in the hospital, this can create emotional
  stress for you. Premature babies may require more
  time, more care and more visits to your pediatrician.

- An added stress is that you have two or more of
  everything—diapers to change, babies to feed,
  clothes to wash, little bodies to bathe, hold and love.

- It's important to ask for help from your partner,
  family and friends. Don't be shy about this. Many
  people are happy to help and are just waiting for
  you to ask.

- As you recover and the babies grow a little older and
  get on some kind of schedule, life will go more
  smoothly.

- Be sure you get enough rest. Your body needs time to recover—probably even more time than if you only had one baby. Be kind to yourself. You'll be glad you did.

Feeding More than One Baby

- One of the greatest challenges for parents of multiples is deciding how to feed them.
- Some mothers want to breastfeed exclusively. (It's an added bonus for multiples because they are usually smaller than single-birth babies, and breast milk is extremely beneficial for them.)
- Some moms say bottlefeeding is the only way to go.
- Others try to combine the two, and breastfeed *and* bottlefeed their babies.
- Breastfeeding your babies, even if it's only for one or two feedings a day, gives them the protection from infection that breast milk provides. Research has shown that even the smallest dose of breast milk gives a baby an advantage over babies fed only formula.
- One of the best things you can do is to consult a lactation specialist—you're going to need some sound advice. You might want to do this *before* the babies are born so you can make a plan.

- If your babies arrive early, and you can't nurse them, begin pumping! This will help stimulate your milk production. Pump from day one, and store your breast milk for the time your babies are able to receive it.
- Pumping tells the body to produce breast milk; it just takes some time.
- Breastfeeding multiples is a challenge. If you decide to try it, experiment with various situations and positions to find what works best for you.
- Some mothers master the art of nursing two babies at the same time. There are special cushions on the market designed to help you do this.
- Switch babies from one breast to the other at different feedings. This ensures each baby gets visual stimulation on both sides. It also helps prevent problems for you, such as engorgement in one breast if one baby isn't feeding as well as the other. By switching breasts, the demand for milk remains about the same for each breast, so breasts tend to remain of equal size.
- Supplementing with formula allows your partner and others to help you feed the babies. You can breastfeed one while someone else bottlefeeds the other.
- Or you can nurse each one for a time, then finish the feeding with formula. In either case, someone else can help you feed the babies.

- Be sure to take good care of yourself. Your attempts at breastfeeding may make you feel like a 24-hour fast-food restaurant, but you'll be giving your babies the best start in life.
- One goal to work toward is getting both babies on the same schedule.
- One baby may be more interested in feeding than the other, but try to feed them both at the same time, when possible.
- Getting your babies to nap and sleep at night at the same time also allows you some rest or free time.

Extra Help after the Babies Are Born

- Even the most efficient woman discovers having more than one baby can be exhausting. Extra help can make a tremendous difference in everyone's life.
- Your time of greatest need is immediately after your babies are born. Ask for help from family, neighbors and friends for the first 4 to 6 weeks after you bring your babies home.
- You may be fairly exhausted yourself, so it's very helpful to have extra pairs of hands available until you all settle into a routine.
- Consider hiring someone to come in for the first few weeks or months to help you out.

- Caring for more than one baby is draining; you'll need time and help, but you will soon discover efficient ways to care for your babies and take care of yourself.
- Having someone available at night can be especially convenient.
- If you cannot afford help, ask a relative who is able to come for a long stay to consider an extended visit to help you get back on your feet.

Postpartum Warning Signs

- If you take good care of yourself after delivery, you should not feel ill. However, occasionally problems do occur.
- Refer to the list of symptoms and warning signs below. Call your doctor immediately if you experience:
    - ~ unusually heavy or sudden increase in vaginal bleeding (more than your normal menstrual flow or soaking more than two sanitary pads in 30 minutes)
    - ~ a vaginal discharge with a strong, unpleasant odor
    - ~ a temperature of 101F or more, except in the first 24 hours after birth
    - ~ chills

~ breasts that are painful or red
~ loss of appetite for an extended period
~ pain, tenderness, redness or swelling in the legs
~ pain in the lower abdomen or in the back
~ painful urination or feeling an intense need to urinate
~ severe pain in the vagina or perineum

Recovering from Your Babies' Births

Recovering from a Vaginal Birth

- Recovery from a vaginal delivery of twins is similar to any other recovery from pregnancy. Discuss the situation with your doctor, and read our other pregnancy books.
- The main difference in your recovery is that you will have more babies to care for. You may need extra sleep, and it is always helpful to have help from friends and family members. You may even consider hiring outside help for the first month or so.

Recovering from a Cesarean Birth

- Recovery from a Cesarean delivery is different from recovery from a vaginal birth.
- You have undergone major abdominal surgery, so be prepared to take it easy for a while.

The Good, the Bad and the Snuggly

"At 42, I was an older first-time pregnant mom. I wasn't ready to be called 'an elderly primip,' the medical term that applies to me. That was 5 years ago, and my two little boys are healthy and happy. But I can still remember the hollow feeling deep inside of me the day we got the results of the twins' amniocentesis. Because of my age and twin pregnancy, my partner and I agreed to genetic amniocentesis at 18 weeks. I really never expected anything to be wrong. However, the test indicated one normal male fetus and one male fetus with Down syndrome. Serious discussions followed with talks about termination of pregnancy and what could be expected for our family and our unborn sons. The genetic counselors were terrific. They helped us come to a decision, which we have never regretted." —*Ellie*

- The nurses and your doctor will go over any precautions before you go home. These should include instructions about normal bleeding and what to do about pain.
- Infection of a Cesarean incision usually occurs 4 to 6 days after surgery.
- If any of the following signs appear, contact your doctor immediately. Signs of infection include:
  - ~ redness that spreads from the edges of the incision
  - ~ fever
  - ~ hardness around the incision
  - ~ discharge from the incision site

- Most doctors recommend you wait to get the go-ahead at your 6-week postpartum checkup before you begin any strenuous activity, start exercising or become sexually active again.
- You can probably resume full activity after your 6-week postpartum checkup, if all is well.

Your Emotions

- Temporary emotional changes are not uncommon during the postpartum period.
- You may have mood swings, mild distress or bouts of crying. See also the discussion of *postpartum distress syndrome (PPDS)* that begins on page 142.
- Mood changes are often a result of birth-associated hormonal changes in your body.
- Lack of sleep may also play a part in how you feel.
- Many women are surprised by how tired they are emotionally and physically in the first few months after the birth of their babies.
- Be sure to take time for yourself, and allow yourself a period of adjustment.
- Sleep and rest are essential after your babies' birth.
- To get the rest you need, go to bed early when possible.
- Take a nap or rest when your babies sleep.

- Ask for help from your partner, family and friends.

Postpartum Distress Syndrome (PPDS)

After your babies are born, you may feel very emotional. This is called *postpartum distress syndrome (PPDS)*. Most women experience some degree of postpartum distress.

- Many experts consider some degree of postpartum distress to be normal.
- Up to 80% of all women have "baby blues." See the discussion on *Different Degrees of Depression* below.
- Baby blues usually appear between 2 days and 2 weeks after the babies' birth.
- They are temporary and usually leave as quickly as they come.
- Symptoms of postpartum depression may not appear until several months *after* delivery.
- Treatment may relieve symptoms in a matter of weeks, and improvement should be significant within 6 to 8 months.
- Often medication is necessary for complete recovery.

Different Degrees of Depression

- The mildest form of postpartum distress is *baby blues.* This situation lasts only a couple of weeks, and symptoms do not worsen.

- A more serious version of postpartum distress is called *postpartum depression (PPD)*. It affects about 10% of all new mothers.
- The difference between baby blues and postpartum depression lies in the frequency, intensity and duration of the symptoms.
- PPD can occur from 2 weeks to 1 year after the birth.
- The most serious form of postpartum distress is *postpartum psychosis (PPP)*. With PPP, the woman may have hallucinations, think about suicide or try to harm the baby.
- Many women who develop postpartum psychosis also exhibit signs of bipolar mood disorder, which is unrelated to childbirth.
- After you give birth, if you believe you are suffering from some form of postpartum distress syndrome, contact your doctor.
- Every postpartum reaction, whether mild or severe, is usually temporary and treatable.

Causes of Postpartum Distress Syndrome

- Researchers aren't sure what causes postpartum distress; not all women experience it. A woman's individual sensitivity to hormonal changes may be part of the cause; the drop in estrogen and progesterone after delivery may contribute to postpartum distress syndrome.

- With multiples, you are more likely to suffer PPD due to your increased responsibility; more demands on your time, which could lead to less sleep; and recovery from a more difficult pregnancy.
- You may also experience greater hormone changes following the delivery of multiples, which could lead to emotional ups and downs.
- Other possible factors include a family history of depression, lack of familial support after the birth, isolation and chronic fatigue.

Handling the Problem

- One of the most important ways you can help yourself is to have a good support system near at hand. Ask family members and friends to help. Ask your husband to take some work leave, or hire someone to come in and help each day.
- Rest when your babies sleep.
- Find other mothers who are in the same situation; it helps to share your feelings and experiences.
- Do some form of moderate exercise every day, even if it's just going for a walk.
- Eat nutritiously, and drink plenty of fluids.

- Go out every day.
- Talk to your doctor about temporarily using antidepressants if the above steps don't work for you.
- Beyond the relatively minor symptoms of baby blues, there are two main forms that postpartum distress syndrome can take: sadness and/or anxiety.
- Some women experience acute depression that can last for weeks or months; they cannot sleep or eat, they feel worthless and isolated, they are sad and they cry a great deal.
- Other women are extremely anxious, restless and agitated. Their heart rate increases.
- Some unfortunate women experience both sets of symptoms at the same time.
- If you experience any symptoms, call your doctor immediately.
- He or she may want to see you in the office, then prescribe a course of treatment for you.

If Your Babies Are Premature

If you are carrying more than one baby, there is a fairly high chance that your babies will be born prematurely. About 50% of all twins deliver before their due date, and nearly all higher-order birth numbers deliver early. Because of the high rate of premature births, we discuss in some depth what you may face if your babies are born early.

- If your babies are born prematurely, you may not be prepared for the event. You may feel sad if you go home without your babies. You may be angry that everything didn't turn out perfectly.
- Don't be too hard on yourself or your partner. Be thankful your babies can be cared for so they will get a good start in life.

Care for Your Babies

- Babies born prematurely are often called *preemies.* The type of care a preemie receives depends on how early he or she was born.
- Some babies are not extremely early, and they won't require the extensive care other babies will. Babies born closer to term may need some stabilization before they are moved to the infant nursery, but they are often soon on their way to going home.
- Other babies need extensive care and will not be able to go home for weeks or months.
- The rule of thumb is that the earlier a baby is born, the longer he or she may need care.

The Good, the Bad and the Snuggly

"It was just like on TV. Earl and I were excited to have an ultrasound and find out if our family would begin with a boy or a girl. I think we each secretly thought we knew beforehand; I knew it was a girl, he was sure of a boy. As the ultrasound exam began and two hearts could be seen beating, it took us a few seconds to get it. We were looking at our twins, one of each sex. Of course we were excited, thrilled and scared, but for different reasons. I was concerned about carrying twins and taking care of them. I think Earl had financial concerns on his mind." —*Teena*

- All premature babies are individuals. Your babies will be evaluated and tended to based on their unique needs.

Immediate Care for Your Newborns

- A preemie needs more care than a full-term baby; much of the care is necessary because a baby's body cannot take over and perform some normal body functions.
- If a preemie is having difficulty breathing, the nursing staff will help the baby with his or her breathing, which can be done in many ways. Immediately after delivery, your baby may be helped in any of the following ways.

- A hood (a large translucent plastic box) may be placed over baby's head to provide additional oxygen if it is needed.
- A bag and mask may be used if a baby is not breathing on his or her own.
- A continuous positive airway pressure (CPAP; pronounced *CEE-pap*) device may be used. It is a two-pronged tube that fits in a baby's nose to provide uninterrupted pressure to his or her lungs.
- A dose of surfactant may be administered to help baby's lungs work more effectively.
- An umbilical artery catheter (UAC) may be inserted into an artery in the umbilicus (umbilical-cord site) to measure blood pressure, to take blood samples and to give medications.
- An I.V. may be inserted into a vein for administration of medication.
- An endo-tracheal (ET) tube may be placed if baby needs to be on a ventilator.
- After each baby is tended to in the delivery room, he or she will be moved to the infant care nursery or to a special neonatal care unit for further treatment, evaluation and care. See *Your Babies' First "Home"* (page 149) and the sections that follow it.
- You may find your babies together in one crib, if they are stable and doing well. Research has found

that keeping twins and triplets together may lead to improved vital signs and shorter hospital stays.

Your Babies' First "Home"

- If any of your babies needs wide-ranging, in-depth care, they will be moved to the neonatal intensive-care unit, also called the NICU (pronounced *NICK-U*).
- If your hospital does not have this special unit, your babies may be transferred to another hospital that has a NICU and services to care for them.
- The nurses and physicians who work in these units have received specialized education and training so they may care for preemies.
- A *neonatologist* is a pediatrician who specializes in diagnosis and treatment of problems in newborns.
- *Neonatal nurses* are registered nurses (RNs) who have received additional, special training in caring for premature and high-risk newborns. You will meet these professionals in the NICU.
- In addition, you may also meet and work with pediatric nutrition specialists, lactation consultants, neonatal respiratory therapists and social workers. All are there to help you and your babies.
- In a NICU, *primary care* is often the norm. With this type of care, one nurse routinely takes care of one

baby. Each nurse will discuss each individual baby's care plan with you and answer your questions. A primary nurse is usually assigned to each baby for each shift.

- If you cannot be at the hospital all the time due to other responsibilities, distance or some other factor, call the NICU to check on your babies. Most NICU staffs welcome your questions.

- You may hesitate to call the NICU nurses because you believe you are bothering them. However, in most cases, they encourage parents to be involved and to contact them. Ask about it at one of your visits to your babies.

Seeing Your Babies for the First Time

- The first time you see your babies for any length of time may be after they have been moved to the NICU.

- You may be overwhelmed when you see them. All the monitors and equipment can be scary and intimidating. However, be assured that all the equipment being used helps give your babies what they need to grow and to continue to develop.

- You may be amazed by the size of your babies. The earlier they are born, the smaller they will be.

- Most preemies don't have much fat on their bodies—a baby usually gains fat during the last few weeks of pregnancy. When babies come early, they haven't had a chance to gain this extra weight. They're not as plump and round as full-term babies.
- Without the fat, they will need help staying warm. Your babies may each be in a warmer, or *isolette,* to help them maintain body temperature. They may be unclothed, without blankets, so the nurses can watch their breathing and body movements more closely.
- Your babies may have a lot more body hair than you expected. This is called *lanugo.*
- Their skin may look thin and fragile, and it may be wrinkled. Wrinkling is due to the fact that they have not gained much fat.

Become Involved with Your Babies

- As soon as you are able to visit the NICU and spend time with your babies, personnel will encourage you to become physically involved with them. In the early days, you may not be able to hold your babies, but you may be able to touch them or to stroke them gently. Lots of contact with your babies helps them grow and thrive.

- As time passes and your babies mature, you will probably be able to hold each one. You will also be encouraged to care for them, such as changing and feeding them. For more on feeding your babies, see the discussion on page 157 *Feeding Your Preemies in the Hospital.*
- When you are with your babies, talk to them softly. You may be surprised how quickly they will come to recognize your voice and respond to you. Your love and attention are important to your babies' physical development and growth.

Massage for Preemies

- In various cultures, vigorous massage is common for a newborn. Some researchers believe these babies develop certain abilities at an earlier age than usual because massage is a part of their daily routine.
- Massage stimulates respiration, circulation, digestion and elimination, and it helps babies sleep more soundly.
- Experts believe massage relieves gas and colic, and it also helps the healing process by easing congestion and pain.
- For a premature baby, medical experts believe massage therapy can help in many ways.
- Studies show that nearly 75% of preemies who were massaged gained more weight and performed better

with developmental tasks. One study showed that massaged infants gained nearly 50% more weight than those who were not massaged.

- Babies who were massaged were also awake and active for longer periods. They scored better on various scales and left the hospital 6 days sooner than babies who were not massaged!
- If you find this technique interesting and want to try it with your babies, talk to the nurses in the NICU. They will know various techniques to use and can suggest what might work best for your babies.

Kangaroo Care

- When you are able to hold your babies, the nurses may encourage you to offer *kangaroo care.*
- Kangaroo care is skin-to-skin contact that is good for a baby in many ways. This technique is very effective in keeping a baby's body temperature normal.
- Studies show that a mother's body temperature adjusts to keep a baby's temperature at the correct point.
- Baby's breathing also becomes more even, and his or her heart rate and blood oxygen levels remain steady, when held in the kangaroo position.
- You are encouraged to hold your unclothed baby (he or she will have a diaper on) against your bare

The Good, the Bad and the Snuggly

"It took a long time for Bill and me to understand how one of our babies could disappear during the pregnancy. At 10 weeks, I had threatened to miscarry and had an ultrasound that revealed twins. We were pretty excited. The bleeding stopped, and I didn't miscarry. A follow-up ultrasound at 18 weeks showed one healthy baby. At first I was mad and wanted to know who had messed up my test. That's when my doctor explained to me what a 'vanishing twin' was. She told me that in 20% of all twin pregnancies, one of the embryos or fetuses dies early in pregnancy and the tissue is reabsorbed. She said no one knows why this happens and there is nothing I did wrong to cause it or anything I could have done to prevent it. A few months later I delivered a beautiful, healthy girl with no sign of the vanishing twin." —*Shayanne*

chest. The personnel in the NICU can offer you some sort of privacy in which to do this.

- Both mom and dad can offer this care. This type of contact helps you both bond with your babies.
- Kangaroo care has been shown to improve parenting abilities because parents become more attuned to their babies' cues.
- Kangaroo care is also very important for your babies' development. Studies show that premature babies who are held this way for an hour or more

every day were more alert and maintained eye contact better as they matured.

Inside the NICU

- You'll see many pieces of equipment and various machines in the NICU. All are there to help provide the best care possible for your babies.
- Monitors record information, ventilators help a baby breathe, lights warm baby or help treat jaundice. Even baby's bed may be unique.
- Equipment in the NICU is made specially for premature babies to take care of their special needs. For example, ventilators provide a smaller volume of air with each breath for a preemie's small lungs. Beds may contain radiant warmers to help maintain a baby's body temperature.
- NICUs provide constant monitoring and round-the-clock care. They are the best chance preemies have to develop and to grow so that they can be released from the hospital and go home.
- The neonatologist and NICU nurses will determine what kind of care and treatment your babies need, including the type of equipment that will best help them.

- Various pieces of NICU equipment and what each is used for include:
  - ~ ventilator—machine that helps a baby breathe through a tube inserted into his or her throat
  - ~ blood-pressure monitor—a small inflatable cuff attached to a baby's arm to record blood pressure
  - ~ cardiorespiratory monitors—sensors that keep track of a baby's breathing and heart rate
  - ~ oxygen saturation monitor or pulse oximeter—sensor that monitors the amount of oxygen in a baby's blood, attached to the foot or hand
  - ~ feeding tube—plastic tube passed through the nose or mouth to help a baby feed
  - ~ overhead warmer—lights mounted overhead or on portable stands, used to keep a baby warm
  - ~ temperature monitor—sensor attached to a baby to measure body temperature
  - ~ bilirubin lights—lights for phototherapy, used to treat jaundice
  - ~ I.V. lines and/or pumps—intravenous lines placed in a baby's veins to deliver medication, nutrients or liquids
  - ~ snugglies—device used to maintain fetal position and make an infant comfortable

~ umbilical-artery catheter—catheter inserted into an artery in the umbilicus (umbilical-cord site) to measure blood pressure, take blood samples and give medications

Feeding Your Preemies in the Hospital

- Feeding is very important for a premature baby. In fact, a baby being able to feed on his own for all of his feedings may be one of the milestones a baby's doctor looks for when considering when to release a baby from the hospital.
- Premature babies often have digestive problems.
- They need to be fed small amounts at a feeding, so they must be fed often.
- Special preemie bottles and nipples must be used.
- Babies tire easily, and they need to learn to suck or to practice sucking.
- Feeding your preemies may be a time-consuming task, but it's worth it when you see them begin to grow.
- For the first few days or weeks after birth, a premature baby is most often fed intravenously for two reasons. The first is that a preemie often does not have the ability to suck and to swallow and therefore cannot

breastfeed or bottlefeed. Second, his or her gastrointestinal system is too immature to absorb nutrients.
- Feeding a preemie by I.V. supplies the needed nutrition in a form he or she can digest.

Tube Feeding

- When a baby matures somewhat, the I.V. feedings
will cease and a feeding tube may be inserted.
- The feeding tube is used until the baby gains enough
strength and maturity to nurse or to take a bottle.
- Tube feeding is often called *gavage feeding.*
- Tubes are made of soft, pliable plastic. Different
types of tubes have been designed to deliver food by
various pathways directly to a baby's tummy or
upper intestine.
- Tube feeding may be continuous or intermittent,
using a gravity drip every 1 to 3 hours.
- Each tube has its own name, which indicates the
route and the destination. Different types include:
  - ~ OG tube—this tube goes through the mouth,
  down the esophagus, into baby's tummy
  - ~ NG tube—this tube goes through the nose to the
  stomach
  - ~ OD tube—this tube goes through the mouth to
  the duodenum, the part of the small intestine
  into which baby's stomach empties

> ~ OJ tube—this tube goes through the mouth to the jejunum, which is farther past the duodenum

- A baby who is tube fed receives fortified breast milk or high-calorie preemie formula through the tube.
- Once a baby's gastrointestinal system demonstrates it can absorb nutrients, the amount will be increased, and the baby may also be offered a bottle or given the opportunity to breastfeed.
- The end goal is to have a baby breastfeeding or bottlefeeding for every feeding. This accomplishment is a major one.
- How quickly your babies move from one form of feeding to another depends on their strength, maturity and growth.
- Even a baby able to take some feedings from the breast or bottle may be given supplemental feedings. Preemies tire quickly and may not be able to get all the nourishment they need from the breast or bottle.
- That's why you may see a baby who is feeding from a bottle also has a feeding tube.
- Babies may also be offered a preemie-sized nipple or pacifier. These encourage development of the sucking and swallowing reflexes. They can also help soothe a baby who is fussy.

Breast Milk Is Best for Premature Babies

- Breast milk is the best nutrition for premature babies. It is rich in antibodies and nutrients essential for a baby's well-being. It may also help reduce the risks of infection and SIDS.
- If you are going to breastfeed your babies, you will need to supply breast milk for that purpose.
- Pumping may be the answer. Studies have shown that any amount of breast milk is beneficial for a preemie, so seriously consider this important task.
- Two nutrients present in breast milk are extremely beneficial to preemies. DHA and ARA are two fatty acids important in baby's brain development and eye development.
- Premature infants miss out on these important nutrients in the womb because they are born early.
- If you cannot breastfeed, ask the NICU nurses if your babies will be fed a special preemie formula that contains these nutrients.
- The composition of your breast milk when your babies are born prematurely is different from the milk when baby is full-term.
- Because of this difference, babies may also be supplemented with formula that contains extra protein, carbohydrates, sodium, folic acid, calcium, iron, phosphorous and vitamins A, D and E.

- These nutrients may be in a form that is easily digested and absorbed by a baby.
- Newborns need calories to regulate body temperature, for energy to grow and to maintain body tissues. Most preemies need about 55 calories per pound of body weight per day.
- If they cannot get all the nutrition they need from breast milk, they may be supplemented with formula developed especially for preemies.

If You Can't Breastfeed

- If you can't breastfeed your babies, there are specialty formulas available.
- One preemie formula by Enfamil contains DHA and ARA. Similac has introduced a formula to use when baby comes home from the hospital. The addition of DHA and ARA appears to help a preemie's visual development.
- You may be advised to use similar formula when you take your babies home.

Problems Some Preemies May Have

When a baby is born prematurely, he or she hasn't had time to finish growing and developing inside the womb.

Being born too early can impact a baby's health in many ways.

- Giving birth to premature babies can be stressful and difficult, but in most cases, things work out fine.
- Many of the problems premature babies encounter pass quickly; some take longer to correct. Some are lifelong.
- Some problems appear rapidly; others develop weeks or months after birth. In some cases, they are not evident until a child starts school.
- With all the medical and technological advances available today, medicine has made many strides forward in the care of premature babies. We are fortunate that many children have few, or no, long-term difficulties.
- Research shows that the earlier a baby is born, the greater the chance he or she will have problems.
- It's not uncommon for extremely premature infants to have more problems than infants who were born later.
- Risks for the very premature infant are still very high. However, researchers continue to explore new ways of treating premature babies and increasing their quality of life.

The Good, the Bad and the Snuggly

"My second pregnancy, the one with twins, was different from the first right from the beginning. My nausea was a lot more severe, and I had to stop taking my prenatal vitamins and every other supplement. Once the nausea improved at 13 weeks, I still didn't feel quite right. I was so tired all the time! For a while I thought it was being pregnant and caring for a 2-year-old. Probably that was part of the problem, but I had forgotten to start taking my vitamins and iron again. My doctor checked for anemia, doing a test called a hematocrit. It was 28, which meant I was severely anemic and needed to do something about it. The doctor explained that anemia can occur gradually and is a lot more likely with multiples. It took a little while, but gradually by taking vitamins and iron and changing my diet, my anemia improved and I felt a lot better. But I still couldn't keep up with my 2-year-old." —*Emma*

- After your babies are discharged from the hospital and you take them home, you may be advised to keep them away from germs as much as possible.
- Their immune systems are immature and need time to develop.
- That may mean staying away from crowds, keeping babies inside and not allowing too many people to hold them.
- You may also be asked to take your babies to the pediatrician weekly for weight checks.

- Your babies may have diverse problems after birth and in the course of life.
- As a premature baby grows, he or she may experience anemia, hearing or vision problems, feeding and growth problems, and problems breathing.
- Developmental delays and/or learning disabilities may not become evident for quite a while.
- Some problems are discussed below. Some are short term; others may need to be dealt with for the rest of a child's life.
- Babies have an amazing ability to heal and to improve, so keep a positive attitude.

Jaundice

- Jaundice is a condition in which the liver cannot get rid of bilirubin, the product of used red blood cells. It is more common in premature babies than in full-term babies.
- A premature baby's liver is less mature than a full-term baby's, so often it cannot process bilirubin effectively.
- The bilirubin builds up in a baby's body, turning skin and sclera (the whites of the eyes) a yellow color.

- If a baby has jaundice, he or she may be given pho-totherapy. This means being placed under a biliru-bin light in the NICU or newborn nursery.
- If treated with phototherapy, a baby may have to wear special goggles or eye patches to protect the eyes. Phototherapy may be administered for 7 to 10 days.

Apnea

- Apnea is defined as a pause in breathing. Preemies typically have irregular breathing rhythms. The in-cidence of apnea decreases as gestational age in-creases. (The longer a baby remains inside the uterus, the lower the chances he or she will have apnea.)
- Preemies often breathe in spurts—a period of deep breathing followed by a shorter period of 5- to 10-second pauses. This is called *periodic breathing*.
- Premature infants respond differently to low oxy-gen levels (hypoxia) than mature babies do. The preemie develops apnea rather than increasing respirations.
- If the period of pauses lasts longer than 10 or 15 seconds, a baby is said to be having an *A/B spell. A* is

for apnea (a pause in breathing); *B* is for *bradycardia* (slow heartbeat).

- This apneic episode may trigger alarms on baby's monitoring devices, if he or she is wearing a monitor.
- After an A/B spell, baby's breathing and heart rate often spontaneously return to normal.
- If a baby experiences frequent A/B spells, the neonatologist may prescribe medication to help regulate breathing. He or she may also suggest an apnea monitor for baby to wear or to sleep on at home, if the problem continues.
- *Important note:* A baby that is at risk for apnea should always sleep in his or her own crib or bassinet. Do not allow baby to sleep with you or to sleep in a family bed!

Anemia

- Anemia is common among preemies.
- A premature baby may not have enough red blood cells to carry oxygen to all of his or her body tissues.
- Your baby may receive vitamins and iron to deal with the problem.
- With severe anemia, blood transfusions may be necessary.

Respiratory Distress Syndrome (RDS)

- *Respiratory distress syndrome (RDS)* is a breathing problem caused by immature lungs in a premature baby.
- In the past, this condition was called *hyaline-membrane disease.* Premature lungs lack surfactant, which gives them the elastic qualities needed for easy breathing.
- Doctors are able to diagnose RDS shortly after birth. Diagnosis is based on a chest X-ray and how much trouble a baby is having breathing.
- Treatment includes supplemental breaths.
- A baby with RDS is often put on a ventilator, also called a *respirator,* that provides these extra breaths.
- Some babies also need CPAP. With CPAP, a plastic tube is fitted into the baby's nostrils to provide pressure to keep tiny air sacs in the lungs inflated.
- If your baby has RDS, he or she will be monitored very closely.
- Baby will probably wear an oximeter or saturation monitor to indicate the level of oxygen in the blood.
- Frequent blood tests to measure carbon dioxide, oxygen and pH blood levels may be done to determine

The Good, the Bad and the Snuggly

"I like to say, 'I delivered an 18-pound baby!' It gets people's attention, but really it was 3 babies that each weighed 6 pounds. During my pregnancy with the triplets, I gained weight so fast that by 30 weeks I felt as big as a cruise ship. I tipped the scales at 185 pounds the visit before I delivered. OK, maybe it was closer to 195, but a year later I was within 5 pounds of my prepregnancy weight. Can you imagine carrying and delivering an 18-pound baby?" —*Ingrid*

how well he or she is breathing. These tests will indicate whether any changes are necessary.

- Prevention of RDS is often one of the main goals in stopping premature labor and delivery.
- If premature labor cannot be stopped, steroids (corticosteroids, betamethasone) may be given before delivery to stimulate fetal lung production of surfactant.
- To be effective, this therapy requires multiple doses for at least 48 hours.
- Following delivery, RDS may be prevented or reduced by delivering synthetic or natural surfactant into the lungs.
- Additional treatment can involve oxygen therapy and help with breathing through the use of a ventilator.

Broncho-Pulmonary Dysplasia (BPD)

- If a baby requires a ventilator or supplemental oxygen a month after birth, he is considered to have *broncho-pulmonary dysplasia (BPD)*.
- Medication may be used to help with breathing.
- Baby may also need supplemental oxygen for a prolonged time.
- If your baby has BPD, take care to keep him from being exposed to germs. If baby develops a bad cold or pneumonia, he or she may need a ventilator.
- A baby with BPD may need supplemental oxygen at home, especially if you live at a high altitude.
- As baby grows and matures, breathing should become easier. However, children who experienced BPD early in life may be more prone to asthma and episodes of wheezing.

Undescended Testicles

- The incidence of undescended testicles is higher in premature baby boys than it is in full-term baby boys.
- Testicles normally descend about 2 months before birth.

- If a baby is born before that time (before 32 weeks of gestation), his testicles may not have descended.
- If this occurs, hormones may be used to bring the testicles into place.
- If a testicle has not descended by the time baby is 15 months old, surgery may be required. Left untreated, the condition can cause infertility.

Patent Ductus Arteriosus (PDA)

- Before birth, a baby doesn't use his or her lungs in the womb to get oxygen, so a blood vessel, called the *ductus arteriosus*, reroutes blood away from the lung.
- Inside the uterus, fetal lungs move in and out; this is called *fetal breathing.* Amniotic fluid moves in and out of the lungs during this process.
- In addition, the fetus manufactures a chemical called *prostaglandin E,* which helps keep the ductus arteriosus open.
- At birth, levels of prostaglandin E drop, the ductus arteriosus closes and blood is sent to the lungs.
- In a premature baby, levels of prostaglandin E may not drop, and the baby continues to produce it. This keeps the ductus arteriosus open, which can cause

breathing difficulties. The condition is called *patent ductus arteriosus (PDA)*.

- Your doctor may treat your baby with medication to stop the production of prostaglandin E. If medication does not work, surgery may be required.

Intracranial Hemorrhage (ICH)

- A baby born earlier than 34 weeks of gestation is at greater risk for bleeding into the brain. This is called *intracranial hemorrhage (ICH)* or *intraventricular hemorrhage (IVH)*.
- The earlier a baby is born, the higher the risk.
- Babies with ICH or IVH are at risk for developing problems later in life, such as cerebral palsy, spasticity and mental retardation.
- Bleeding most often occurs within the first 72 hours after birth. Ultrasound is used to examine the baby's head to determine if bleeding has occurred.
- If an episode of ICH or IVH is mild, no treatment is necessary. Baby will be observed closely by those in the NICU.
- For more severe cases, treatment will be ordered. The type of treatment will be determined by your physician.

Retinopathy of Prematurity (ROP)

- Fifty years ago, some very premature babies who survived had severe vision impairment; some were even blind. The problem was called *retrolental fibroplasia.*
- It was believed to be caused by the use of oxygen.
- Today, we have a better understanding of the problem and now call it *retinopathy of prematurity (ROP).* The problem is most common in very premature babies.
- It's uncommon for babies born after 33 or 34 weeks of gestation to have it.
- When a baby is born early, retinal development of the eye is incomplete.
- ROP occurs when the delicate retina development is disturbed because baby is born too early.
- If personnel in the NICU believe your baby may be at risk for ROP, an ophthalmologist who specializes in premature babies can examine baby after he or she is 6 weeks old.
- Most cases of ROP are mild and resolve on their own. If the problem is more severe, treatment with cryotherapy may be necessary.
- We are fortunate that retinal detachment and blindness are uncommon today. ROP mainly affects only the very smallest, unstable preemies.

Respiratory Syncytial Virus (RSV)

- *Respiratory syncytial virus (RSV)* often begins as a cold; it can develop into pneumonia or bronchiolitis.
- The problem can arise quickly, so call your pediatrician immediately if your baby develops wheezing and/or rapid breathing with a cold.
- Because there is no medication available to treat the problem, prevention is key.
- Keep baby away from crowds, and wash your hands frequently during the cold season (winter and early spring).
- In addition, talk with your pediatrician about protective immunizations.

Development of Your Premature Babies

- In some ways, a premature baby is a smaller version of a full-term baby.
- But in other ways, a preemie is *very* different.
- Premature infants live in a world that is different from the womb and also different from the life of a full-term infant at home.
- Preemies are unique—they require special attention and treatment.

- And *your* preemies are unique in their own right!
- Never compare your babies to other children, even another premature baby.
- They will grow and develop at their own pace.
- It's helpful to consider their due date the point from which development actually begins.
- Think of the time between their actual birth date and their predicted due date as "catch-up time."
- This period of time allows your babies to finish growing and maturing as if they had still been in your womb.
- Their due date is the point from which to gauge growth and progress.
- *Note:* When we speak of a "young preemie" in this section, we are talking about a baby born earlier in pregnancy. Although we cannot give an exact time frame, a young preemie refers to a child born between 24 and 31 weeks of gestation.

Your Babies' Overall Development

- A premature baby doesn't act like a full-term baby.
- To help you understand why there is such a difference, it's helpful to know how babies develop.
- Every baby has five important areas of development— they are all controlled by the brain and develop together. The five developmental areas are:

The Good, the Bad and the Snuggly

"When she first offered the test to me, I thought my doctor was planning on doing a test only done on women carrying triplets. It was called a *triple screen*. The test measures three blood components in pregnant women and can be helpful in predicting Down syndrome during pregnancy. However, the test is a lot more useful when you are only carrying one baby, not three. She said that with multiple pregnancies it is difficult to know what normal values are for the triple screen, and most of the time multiple pregnancies are followed with ultrasound and sometimes an amniocentesis. I also learned that there is a *quad screen* that adds another blood test, for a total of four. This test is not as useful in multiple pregnancies as it is with only one baby." —*Petula*

- ~ physiological—bodily functions that happen automatically, such as heart rate, breathing, digestion and elimination
- ~ motor—body movements, muscle tone
- ~ states of consciousness—sleeping and wakefulness, and the change from one to another
- ~ attention—being able to focus
- ~ self-regulation—keeping the other four areas in balance
- The nervous system of a premature baby is not as mature or as developed as that of a full-term baby. This can affect a preemie in many different ways.
- Some of the things you may see with immature development include:

~ immature physiological development—baby gags easily, has an uneven heart rate, breathes unevenly or changes color often

~ immature motor development—baby twitches, tenses or trembles, is limp or doesn't stay curled up

~ immature control of states of consciousness—baby doesn't stay alert for long, fusses a lot

~ immature development of attention—baby can't focus on you, tires easily when trying to respond

~ immature self regulation—baby has difficulty calming down, cannot deal with many things going on at the same time

- A baby's hearing is fairly well developed by 20 weeks of gestation. He can hear inside the womb, so even when he is born early he will be able to hear.

- Sight takes longer to develop. Preemies take longer to focus on an object than full-term babies. Vision is not as clear for a preemie either.

The Sleep/Wake States of Preemies

- Sleep states for a baby are different from that of an adult.

- Babies have two distinct sleep patterns, three wake states and an in-between sleep-and-wake state.

- All babies go to sleep in light sleep, and if they aren't disturbed, wake from a light sleep.

- The various sleep and wake states are discussed below.
  - ~ Deep sleep (non-REM sleep)—In this state, baby is motionless. Occasionally he will sigh or twitch. Breathing is even. This type of sleep is important for baby's growth. A full-term baby spends about 15 to 20 minutes in deep sleep and 65 to 70 minutes in light sleep. Young preemies have very little deep sleep; they may move more, and breathing may be uneven. A young preemie may spend only a few minutes in deep sleep before moving back into light sleep.
  - ~ Light sleep (REM sleep)—During this state, baby may move a lot and make noises. Breathing is uneven, and eyelids may open and close. This is called *rapid eye movement (REM).* Young preemies spend most of their time in light sleep.
  - ~ Wake states—Babies have several levels of wakefulness, including drowsy, actively awake and alert. When baby is *drowsy,* he has trouble staying awake or waking up; he doesn't move much. When he is *actively awake,* he's awake but not looking at anything; he may be quite active. When he is *alert,* his eyes are wide open, and he looks around. Preemies may try to focus, but their eyes are not wide open, and they do not seem fully alert.
  - ~ Sleep-wake transition—It's hard to determine if a baby is in this state. A baby may actually wake a

little then go back into light sleep several times before finally waking up. Young preemies may be in this state quite often.

- If a baby is born before 26 or 27 weeks, it may be difficult to determine if he is awake. There is no alert state.

- When birth is between 27 and 30 weeks, a preemie may be alert for a short time only. When he is awake, he may be drowsy or actively awake.

- As baby grows, the amount of time he spends in an alert state increases.

- The alert state is important because baby must be alert to focus on, and pay attention to, what he sees. This is an important function of learning.

- Research has shown that even when a preemie is 39 to 40 weeks old, he is not alert as often as a full-term baby.

Reaching Milestones

- A baby born early may take longer to reach an event marking a significant new development or stage.

- These are called *milestones*. Being familiar with expected milestones will help you determine how your baby is progressing.

- It really doesn't matter *when* a child reaches a milestone as long as he or she eventually reaches it!
- When you evaluate how your children are developing, correct their age for the weeks of prematurity. Consider developmental age from the actual due date, not the date of birth! For example, if your babies were born on April 18th but their due date was actually June 6th, begin measuring development from June 6th. Consider this your children's "developmental birthday."

You Can Help Your Babies' Development

- We know preemies may face many challenges in their lives as they grow.
- However, research shows that many children who were born prematurely may be on a par with their peers as they get older if their home environment is stimulating and they are offered a great deal of interaction.
- Ways to help your babies are within your control— you *can* make a difference in your children's lives in many ways!
- As parents, you are your babies' most important social partners, whether babies are premature or full term.

- There are many ways you can help your babies in their development.
- It takes patience and attention on your part, but if you make the effort to do the things listed below, you'll help your babies and yourselves.
    - ~ Learn how to assess each baby's behavior. Become familiar with their different moods, and determine what each needs from you.
    - ~ Determine what kind of interaction each baby wants and how you should respond.
    - ~ Create a comfortable environment for your babies by keeping noise levels low, allowing them to sleep when they need it and providing chances for them to interact when they are alert.
    - ~ Acknowledge that your preemies are like no others—allow them the time they need to progress at their own individual rates.
    - ~ Trust your instincts. You know your babies better than anyone else. If something doesn't feel right to you, check it out!

When to Be Concerned

- Most of the time, babies who are born early catch up with their peers, and by the time they are in school, no one would ever know your babies were born prematurely.

- However, sometimes reaching a milestone late can signal a problem for a child. Be concerned when the following occur.
  - ~ Your child is delayed in more than one area. Often a child will slow up in development in one area while concentrating on another. However, if one of your children is not developing in quite a few areas, it's time to be concerned. If you are concerned, discuss it with your pediatrician.
  - ~ Delay is far from the norm. If baby is delayed 3 or 4 months beyond the point at which he or she should be doing something, it's time for concern.
  - ~ Your child doesn't respond when you speak to him or her or doesn't seem to understand. Your baby should be able to follow simple directions at certain ages. By 1 year, baby should be able to point to a favorite toy if you ask where it is. By 15 months, he or she should follow simple requests, such as bringing you the sock when you ask. If your baby doesn't respond, talk with your pediatrician about it.
- If you have questions or concerns about any delays your child is experiencing, it may be time to explore the situation with your pediatrician.

The Good, the Bad and the Snuggly

"I was determined to deliver my twins vaginally. I knew I wouldn't feel like I had experienced the miracle of birth if I had a Cesarean section. I talked to my doctor about it, and he said I was in good enough shape that he would allow me to try to labor and to deliver vaginally if the babies were in the correct birth positions—head down. When I went into labor at 35 weeks, an ultrasound at the hospital showed that both babies were in the correct positions, so he gave me the OK to proceed. But he told me that if either baby was in any kind of danger, he'd have to do a C-section. I was prepared for a vaginal birth; Ben and I had gone to prenatal classes and had practiced the breathing techniques and relaxation exercises for weeks. We were ready!

I labored about 8½ hours and delivered Kelton without too much trouble. I was feeling pretty ecstatic. But then Jeremy began having trouble—something seemed to be wrong with the cord. My doctor told me that he was going to have to do a C-section to deliver him immediately. I had to be put under with general anesthesia, but Jeremy was successfully delivered and was all right. My recovery was a real pain—I had the discomfort of the episiotomy I had with Kelton and the pain of abdominal surgery with Jeremy. It took me a lot longer than I ever imagined to get back on my feet. Thank heavens I had such wonderful people helping me out when I went home." —*Cassie*

- Discuss your concerns with your baby's doctor; he or she will advise you and recommend specialists to provide further medical assessment or treatment.
- During the first year, remember always to consider your babies' "due-date age" as your point of reference for all developmental discussions.

When Babies Go Home

- At some point, you will be able to take your babies home.
- With multiples, you may take them home separately, when each gains sufficient weight and is feeding well enough to leave the hospital.
- It's hard not to be able to take them home together, at the same time. Some babies need more time in the hospital due to complications. However, you can look forward to the day you'll all be together.
- Your babies will be ready to go home when they:
  - ~ have no medical problems that require them to be in the hospital
  - ~ can maintain a stable body temperature
  - ~ can take all of their feedings on their own (no tube feeding)
  - ~ are gaining weight

- Taking babies home can be wonderful, but it may also cause you some concern. Will you be able to meet their needs? Will you be able to care for them?
- The people in the NICU will help you prepare for this important event.
- Many NICUs let you "room in" with baby just before you take the baby home. It's a great opportunity to take care of baby on your own while you have the nursing staff at hand to help.
- The personnel in the NICU can help you plan any special care before you take your babies home. Once home, most preemies do well.
- When you are home, ask your partner to help you and to share the responsibility of parenting.
- Ask for help—and accept it—from others who offer it, including family, friends and neighbors.

Preemie Equipment You May Want to Consider

- Your lives will be different when you take your preemies home. It's not the same as bringing a full-term baby home.
- You may need different equipment, or you may not need some equipment yet.
- Your schedule may be very hectic because you have to feed your babies more often.

- You may have your hands full tending to your babies and any other children you have.
- For babies' first trip home and for future trips in the car, you may want to consider a car bed.
- This device allows a baby to lie flat. This position is often better for preemies because they may have trouble breathing in a normal-size car seat.
- Or you may want to consider Cosco's Ultra Dream Ride, a car bed for preemies as small as 5 pounds. It converts to a rear-facing car seat that you can use until a baby is 20 pounds. See the *Resource Section,* page 187, for further information.
- If you didn't get any preemie pacifiers in the hospital, consider buying some. There are many on the market. This type of pacifier fits a premature baby's tiny mouth more comfortably than a regular pacifier.
- You're going to need preemie diapers. They are designed for premature babies weighing between 1 and 6 pounds.
- Disposable preemie diapers are adjustable (they have an expandable back panel) and have the narrowest crotch of any diaper available to allow for proper leg positioning.
- They are also absorbent and can absorb up to 2½ ounces, or 5 tablespoons, of liquid.

- If you want to use cloth diapers, ask at the hospital about where you can purchase them.
- If you are planning to use a diaper service, call the company and ask if they supply preemie diapers.
- Your babies' nursery can be set up almost any-where—it may be a separate bedroom or an alcove or area in your bedroom. Babies can sleep just about anywhere—in a cradle, a bassinet or a crib.
- The most essential pieces of equipment you need when you bring your babies home are a place for them to sleep and a place for diaper changing and dressing.
- Your babies don't need much to wear when they are very small. It may be difficult to find clothes that fit them. Diapers, T-shirts, gowns that open at the bottom, footed sleepers and socks are often enough to get you started.
- Be sure you have plenty of warm blankets; if your babies are premature, they may have trouble regulating their body temperatures.

Resources

General Information for Parents

For Adoptive Parents
Good resource for adoption information
www.adoption.com

American Academy of Family
Practitioners (AAFP)
www.aafp.com

American Academy of Pediatrics
(AAP)
P.O. Box 927, Dept. C
Elk Grove Village, IL 60009-0927
www.aap.org

American College of Obstetricians
and Gynecologists (ACOG)
P.O. Box 4500
Kearneysville, WV 25430
800-762-2264
www.acog.com

American Psychological Association
(APA)
202-336-5700
www.apa.org

Car-Seat Installation
877-FIT-4-A-KID
www.fitforakid.com

Centers for Disease Control
*For up-to-date information on many
medical issues*
www.cdc.gov

Child Care Aware
800-424-2246

ChildrenFirst, Inc.
800-244-5317
www.childrenfirst.com

Children's Defense Fund
www.childrensdefense.org

COPE
37 Clarendon St.
Boston, MA 02116
617-357-5588

Formulas that Contain DHA and ARA
Nestle Good Start
www.verybestbaby.com
Similac Advance
www.similacadvance.com
Enfamil LIPIL
www.enfamil.com

Homemade Baby-Food Recipes
www.americanbaby.com/babyfood
www.babytalk.com

Intensive-Care Parenting magazine
ICU Parenting
RD #10, Box 176
Brush Creek Rd.
Irwin, PA 15642

Internal Revenue Service
For information on child-care expenses
800-829-1040
www.irs.ustreas.gov

Juvenile Products Manufacturers
Association
*For information on baby products,
  recalls and other pertinent information*
236 Route 38 West, Suite 100
Moorestown, NJ 08057
www.jpma.org

March of Dimes
*For information on various serious
  childhood illnesses and diseases*
888-663-4637
www.modimes.org

Military Families
For families of military personnel
www.4militaryparents.com

National Association for Sick Child
Daycare
205-324-8447
www.nascd.com

National Organization of Single
Mothers
P.O. Box 68
Midland, NC 28107-0068
704-888-KIDS (704-888-5437)

Organic Formulas
*For a listing of stores that carry organic
  formulas*
www.horizonorganic.com

Parent's Resources
P.O. Box 107, Planetarium Sta.
New York, NY 10024
212-866-4776

Poison Control Center (national
hotline)
800-222-1222

Product Recalls
*For the latest baby-product recalls and
  warnings*
www.childrecall.com
www.cpsc.gov
www.jpma.org

Social Security Administration
800-772-1213
www.ssa.gov

Tri-Flow Nipple System
From Munchkin
www.munchkininc.com
800-344-2229

U.S. Consumer Products Safety
Commission
800-638-2772
www.cpsc.gov

Vaccinations
*For information on vaccines from the
  Children's Hospital of Philadelphia*
www.vaccine.chop.edu

Women's Bureau Publications
For summary of state laws on family
leave
U.S. Department of Labor
Women's Bureau Clearing House
Box EX
200 Constitution Ave., NW
Washington, DC 20210
800-827-5335
See also www.ecoc.gov/facts/
fs-preg.html

Websites for Further Information
www.americanbaby.com
www.babycenter.com
www.babyzone.com
www.bellycast.com
www.childmagazine.com
www.family.com
www.ibaby.com
www.ivillage.com
www.parenthoodweb.com

Breastfeeding Information

Avent
800-542-8368
www.aventamerica.com

Beechnut Nutrition Hotline
800-523-6633

Best Start
3500 E. Fletcher Ave., Suite 519
Tampa, FL 33613
800-277-4975

Breastfeeding Help
For 24-hour breastfeeding support,
referrals to lactation consultants and
helpful videos
www.breastfeeding.com

FDA Breast Implant Information Line
800-532-4440

FDA Hotline
800-332-4010

International Lactation Consultant
Association
www.ilca.org
919-787-5181

La Leche League International
1400 N. Meacham Rd.
Schaumburg, IL 60173-4840
800-LA-LECHE or check local
telephone directory
www.lalecheleague.org

Medela, Inc.
P.O. Box 660
McHenry, IL 60051
800-TELL-YOU (800-735-5968)

National Center for Nutrition and
Dietetics
Consumer Nutrition Hotline
800-366-1655

National Maternal and Child Health
Clearinghouse
2070 Chain Bridge Rd., Suite 45
Vienna, VA 22182
703-821-8955, ext. 254

Wellstart
4062 First Ave.
San Diego, CA 92103
619-295-5192

Websites for Further Information
www.breastfeedingbasics.com
www.moms4milk.org
www.breastfeed.com

Child Care

Child Care Aware Hotline
800-424-2246

Department of Health and
Human Services
*National Child Care Information
  Center*
800-616-2242

International Nanny Association
800-297-1477
www.nanny.org

National Association for the
Education of Young Children
www.naeyc.org

National Association of Child Care
Resource and Referral Agencies
800-424-2246
202-393-5501
www.childcarerr.org
www.naccrra.net

National Resource Center for Health
and Safety in Child Care
800-598-5437
www.nrc.uchsc.edu

Working Mother
www.workingmother.com

Children's Illnesses and Problems; Children with Special Needs

Arthritis
American Juvenile Arthritis
Organization
1314 Spring St., NW
Atlanta, GA 30309
404-872-7100

Asthma and Allergies
Allergy and Asthma Network
3554 Chain Bridge Rd., Suite 200
Fairfax, VA 22030
800-878-4403

American College of Allergy, Asthma
and Immunology (ACAAI)
*Informative news services for parents
  and patients. Site is maintained by
  allergists and ACAAI*
800-842-7777
allergy.mcg.edu

Asthma & Allergy Foundation of
America
1835 K St., NW, Suite P-900
Washington, DC 20006
202-293-2950

Autism
National Society for Children and
Adults with Autism
1234 Massachusetts Ave.,
NE, Suite 1017
Washington, DC 20005
202-783-0125

Birth Defects
March of Dimes
1275 Mamaroneck Ave.
White Plains, NY 10605
914-428-7100
www.modimes.org

National Maternal and Child Health
Clearinghouse
3520 Prospect St., NW
Washington, DC 20057
202-625-8410

Blindness
American Foundation for the Blind
15 W. 16th St.
New York, NY 10011
212-620-2000

Helen Keller National Center for
Deaf-Blind Youths and Adults
111 Middle Neck Rd.
Sands Point, NY 11050
516-944-8900

Cancer
Association for Research of
Childhood Cancer
P.O. Box 251
Buffalo, NY 14225
716-681-4433

Candlelighters Childhood Cancer
Foundation
1901 Pennsylvania Ave., NW
Suite 1001
Washington, DC 20006
202-659-5136

Cerebral Palsy
National Easter Seal Society
2023 W. Ogden Ave.
Chicago, IL 60612
312-243-8400

United Cerebral Palsy Association
60 E. 34th St.
New York, NY 10016
212-481-2811

Cleft Palate
American Cleft Palate Association
331 Salk Hall
University of Pittsburgh
Pittsburgh, PA 15261
412-681-9620

American Cleft Palate Foundation
1218 Grandview Ave.
Pittsburgh, PA 15211
800-242-5337

Cystic Fibrosis
Cystic Fibrosis Foundation
6000 Executive Blvd., Suite 309
Rockville, MD 20852
301-881-9130

Down Syndrome
Association for Children with Down
Syndrome
2616 Martin Ave.
Bellmore, NY 11710
516-221-4700

National Down Syndrome Society
(NDSS)
666 Broadway
New York, NY 10012-2317
800-221-4602

Epilepsy
Epilepsy Foundation of America
4351 Garden City, Suite 406
Landover, MD 20785
301-459-3700

Food Allergies
Food Allergy and Anaphylaxis
Network
www.foodallergy.org
800-929-4040

Fragile X Syndrome
National Fragile X Foundation
1441 York St., Suite 303
Denver, CO 80206
800-688-8765

Gastrointestinal Disorders
American Digestive Disease Society
7720 Wisconsin Ave.
Bethesda, MD 20014
301-652-9293

General Information
CARESS (Information on services for
parents of children with disabilities)
P.O. Box 1492
Washington, DC 20013-1492
800-695-0285

National Association for Rare
Disorders
P.O. Box 8923
New Fairfield, CT 06182

Hearing Problems
American Society for Deaf Children
814 Thayer Ave.
Silver Spring, MD 20910
301-585-5400

American Speech-Language-Hearing
Association
10801 Rockville Pike
Rockville, MD 20852
301-897-5700

Helen Keller National Center for
Deaf-Blind Youths and Adults
111 Middle Neck Rd.
Sands Point, NY 11050
516-944-8900

Heart Problems
American Heart Association
7272 Greenville Ave.
Dallas, TX 75231-4596
800-242-8721

Congenital Heart Anomalies—
Support, Education, Resources
2112 N. Wilkins Rd.
Swanton, OH 43558
419-825-5575

Hemophilia
National Hemophilia Foundation
19 W. 34th St., Rm. 1204
New York, NY 10001
212-563-0211

World Federation of Hemophilia
Suite 2902
1155 Dorchester Blvd., W.
Montreal, Quebec H3B 2L3 Canada

Leukemia
Leukemia Society of America, Inc.
800 Second Ave.
New York, NY 10017
212-573-8484

Limb Disorders
Cherub Association of Families of
Children with Limb Disorders
936 Delaware Ave.
Buffalo, NY 14209

Liver Disease
Children's Liver Foundation
76 S. Orange Ave., Suite 202
South Orange, NJ 07079
201-761-1111

Mental Retardation (see also
Down Syndrome)
Association for Children with
Retarded Mental Development, Inc.
817 Broadway
New York, NY 10003
212-470-7200

Phenylketonuria
National PKU Foundation
6301 Tejas Dr.
Pasadena, TX 77503
713-487-4802

Psoriasis
National Psoriasis Foundation
6415 SW Canyon Court, Suite 200
Portland, OR 97221
503-297-1545

Reye's Syndrome
National Reye's Syndrome Foundation
426 N. Lewis St.
P.O. Box 829
Bryan, OH 43506
800-233-7393

Respiratory Syncytial Virus (RSV)
RSV Information
www.rsvprotection.com
877-819-9851

Sickle-Cell Disease
National Association for Sickle-Cell
Disease
3460 Wilshire Blvd., Suite 1012
Los Angeles, CA 90010
213-731-1166

Sickle-Cell Disease Association of
America, Inc.
200 Corporate Pt., Suite 495
Culver City, CA 90230
800-421-8453

Spina Bifida
Spina Bifida Association of America
4590 MacArthur Blvd., NW, #250
Washington, DC 20007-4226
800-621-3141

*Sudden Infant Death
Syndrome (SIDS)*
Guild for Infant Survival
P.O. Box 3841
Davenport, IA 52808

National Center for the Prevention of
Sudden Infant Death Syndrome
330 N. Charles St.
Baltimore, MD 21201
301-547-0300

National Sudden Infant Death
Syndrome Clearinghouse
8201 Greensboro Dr., Suite 600
McLean, VA 22102
703-821-8955; 703-625-8410

National Sudden Infant Death
Syndrome Foundation
8240 Professional Place, Suite 205
Landover, MD 20785
301-459-3388; 800-221-7437 (SIDS)

Tay-Sachs Disease
National Tay-Sachs & Allied Disease
Association, Inc.
92 Washington Ave.
Cedarhurst, NY 11516
516-569-4300

Multiples

Center for Loss in Multiple Birth
c/o Jean Kollantai
P.O. Box 1064
Palmer, AK 99645
907-746-6123

Center for Study of Multiple Births
333 E. Superior St., Room 464
Chicago, IL 60611
312-266-9093

Mothers of Supertwins (M.O.S.T.)
(triplets or more)
P.O. Box 951
Brentwood, NY 11717
516-434-MOST
www.mostonline.org

Multiple Birth Resources
70 W. Sylvester Place
Highlands Ranch, CO 80126
888-627-9519
www.expectingmultiples.com

Multiple Births Foundation
Queen Charlotte's and Chelsea
Hospital
Goldhawk Rd.
London, England W6 OXG
081-748-4666, ext. 5201

National Online Fathers of Twins
Club
www.member.aol.com/nofotc

National Organization of Mothers of
Twins Clubs, Inc. (NOMOTC)
P.O. Box 438
Thompson Station, TN 37179-0438
505-275-0955
www.nomotc.org

Triplet Connection
P.O. Box 99571
Stockton, CA 95209
209-474-0885
www.tripletconnection.org

Twin Services
P.O. Box 10066
Berkeley, CA 94709
510-524-0863
twinservices@juno.com

Twin-to-Twin Transfusion Syndrome
(TTTS) Foundation
Mary Slaman-Forsythe, Executive
Director
411 Longbeach Parkway
Bay Village, OH 44140
216-899-8887

Twins Foundation
P.O. Box 6043
Providence, RI 02940-6043
401-729-1000

Twins Hope
*International center for twin-related
 diseases*
www.twinshope.com

Twins Magazine
5350 S. Roslyn St., Suite 400
Englewood, CO 80111
800-328-3211
www.twinsmagazine.com

Twins World
*Good resource for couples expecting
 multiples*
www.twinsworld.com

Premature Infants

Clothing for preemies
www.visitlittleme.com
www.preemie.com
www.gap.com
www.babiesrus.com

Cosco Ultra Dream Ride
Car bed/seat for preemies
www.djgusa.com
800-544-1108

Early Arrivals
www.earlyarrivals.com

ECMO Moms and Dads
c/o Blair and Gayle Wilson
P.O. Box 53848
Lubbock, TX 79453
806-794-0259

Gerber
Preemie pacifiers
www.gerber.com

Intensive-Care Parenting magazine
ICU Parenting
RD #10, Box 176
Brush Creek Rd.
Irwin, PA 15642

Preemie diapers
Pampers
www.pampers.com

800-543-3331
Huggies
www.drugstore.com
800-447-9423

Premature Babies
For information on, and products for,
  premature infants
www.earlyarrivals.com
www.pediatrics.wisc.edu/patientcare/
preemies

Safety for Your Baby

Auto Safety Hotline
888-327-4236

Back to Sleep
P.O. Box 29111
Washington, DC 20040
800-505-2742

Car Seats for Pickup Trucks
Pioneered Safety System from XSCI
800-630-6850

Car-Seat Safety
Child passenger safety
www.childsafety.org

Crib-Sheet Safety
Baby Sleep Safe crib sheet anchor
800-420-1280
Clouds and Stars quick-zip crib sheets
www.cloudsandstars.com
866-325-6837

Danny Foundation
For information on crib dangers
3158 Danville Blvd.
P.O. Box 680
Alamo, CA 94507
800-833-2669

General Motors
"Precious Cargo: Protecting the
 Children Who Ride with
 You" (free booklet)
800-247-9168

International Association of
Chiefs of Police
Operation Kids
800-843-4227

Juvenile Products Manufacturers
Association
236 Route 38 West, Suite 100
Moorestown, NJ 08057
www.jpma.org

National Highway Traffic Safety
Administration
Auto safety hotline
800-424-9393
www.nhtsa.gov

National Lead Information Hotline
and Clearinghouse
800-424-LEAD

National SAFE KIDS Campaign
800-441-1888
www.safekids.org

Safety Alerts
For information on recalls
www.safetyalerts.com

SafetyBeltUSA
123 Manchester Blvd.
Inglewood, CA 90301
800-745-SAFE
www.carseat.org

U.S. Consumer Products Safety
Commission
800-638-2772
www.cpsc.gov

Also by Glade B. Curtis, M.D., M.P.H., OB/GYN and Judith Schuler, M.S.

Your Pregnancy Week by Week, 5th edition
ISBN: 1-55561-346-2 (paper)
1-55561-347-0 (cloth)

Your Pregnancy Journal Week by Week
ISBN: 1-55561-343-8

Your Pregnancy for the Father to Be
ISBN: 0-7382-1002-1

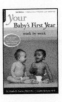

Your Baby's First Year Week by Week,
2nd edition
ISBN: 0-7382-0975-9 (paper)
0-7382-0974-0 (cloth)

Bouncing Back After Your Pregnancy
ISBN: 0-7382-0606-7

Da Capo Lifelong Books are available wherever books are sold and at special discounts for bulk purchases in the U.S. by corporations, institutions, and other organizations. For more information, please contact the Special Markets Department at the Perseus Books Group, 11 Cambridge Center, Cambridge, MA 02142, or call (800) 255-1514, or email special.markets@perseusbooks.com.